THE EVERYTHING® VEGAN WEDDING BOOK

Dear Reader,

Congratulations! You are officially a member of the bride-to-be club . . . the vegan-bride-to-be-club, no less! Make no mistake, any wedding planning is a frenzy of excitement, laughter, tears, and yes, a little bit of stress. But that is all part of planning a wedding, whether or not it is a vegan wedding.

Your vegan fundamentals and beliefs will influence and impact each and every decision. However, you must remember that at its core, a wedding is a wedding. There is a method to this madness. It is your time to take that tried and true planning path and twist, turn, and mold to incorporate your vegan values and personality . . . and there you will find wedding-planning success.

Weddings are an investment of time and money and emotions. Along your chosen planning path, you may be questioned about your decisions, you may find people—even your family or best friend—may not understand. You really need to make a commitment to stay strong, stay on task, stay consistent with your partner, and continue to plan your vegan wedding like the smart, fabulous vegan woman you are.

I have watched hundreds of couples plan their weddings "their way," and I know that with thought and care, you can plan a vegan wedding that wows your guests and leaves them wanting more . . . so get out there and plan, prepare, and take that walk down the aisle in stunning, cruelty-free shoes, as you celebrate your decisions and make no apologies.

Holly Lefevre

Welcome to the EVERYTHING® Series!

These handy, accessible books give you all you need to tackle a difficult project, gain a new hobby, comprehend a fascinating topic, prepare for an exam, or even brush up on something you learned back in school but have since forgotten.

You can choose to read an Everything® book from cover to cover or just pick out the information you want from our four useful boxes: e-questions, e-facts, e-alerts, and e-ssentials.

We give you everything you need to know on the subject, but throw in a lot of fun stuff along the way, too.

We now have more than 400 Everything® books in print, spanning such wide-ranging categories as weddings, pregnancy, cooking, music instruction, foreign language, crafts, pets, New Age, and so much more. When you're done reading them all, you can finally say you know Everything®!

QUESTION

Answers to
common questions

FACT

Important snippets
of information

ALERT

Urgent
warnings

ESSENTIAL

Quick
handy tips

PUBLISHER Karen Cooper

DIRECTOR OF ACQUISITIONS AND INNOVATION Paula Munier

MANAGING EDITOR, EVERYTHING® SERIES Lisa Laing

COPY CHIEF Casey Ebert

ASSISTANT PRODUCTION EDITOR Melanie Cordova

ACQUISITIONS EDITOR Kate Powers

SENIOR DEVELOPMENT EDITOR Brett Palana-Shanahan

EDITORIAL ASSISTANT Ross Weisman

EVERYTHING® SERIES COVER DESIGNER Erin Alexander

LAYOUT DESIGNERS Colleen Cunningham, Elisabeth Lariviere, Ashley Vierra, Denise Wallace

Visit the entire Everything® series at www.everything.com

THE
EVERYTHING®
VEGAN WEDDING
BOOK

From the dress to the cake, all you need to know
to have your wedding your way!

Holly Lefevre

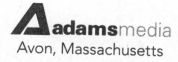

Aadamsmedia
Avon, Massachusetts

To my husband and kiddos for their constant love and support.

An Everything® Series Book.
Everything® and everything.com® are registered trademarks of F+W Media, Inc.

Published by Adams Media, a division of F+W Media, Inc.
57 Littlefield Street, Avon, MA 02322 U.S.A.
www.adamsmedia.com

ISBN 10: 1-4405-2786-5
ISBN 13: 978-1-4405-2786-9
eISBN 10: 1-4405-2845-4
eISBN 13: 978-1-4405-2845-3

Printed in the United States of America.

10 9 8 7 6 5 4 3 2 1

The Everything® Vegan Wedding Book contains material adapted and abridged from: *The Everything® Wedding Book, 4th Edition* by Katie Martin, copyright © 2011 by F+W Media, Inc., ISBN 10: 1-4405-0156-4, ISBN 13: 978-1-4405-0156-2; *The Everything® Green Wedding Book* by Wenona Napolitano, copyright © 2009 by F+W Media, Inc., ISBN 10: 1-59869-811-7, ISBN 13: 978-1-59869-811-4; *The Everything® Wedding Checklist Book, 3rd Edition* by Holly Lefevre, copyright © 2011 by F+W Media, Inc., ISBN 10: 1-4405-0185-8, ISBN 13: 978-14405-0185-2; *The Everything® Wedding Organizer, 2nd Edition* by Shelly Hagen, copyright © 2006 by F+W Media, Inc., ISBN 10: ISBN 13: 978-1-59337-640-6; and *The Everything® Wedding Etiquette Book, 3rd Edition* by Holly Lefevre, copyright © 2010 by F+W Media, Inc., ISBN 10: 1-60550-094-1, ISBN 13: 978-1-60550-094-2.

Library of Congress Cataloging-in-Publication Data
is available from the publisher.

This book is available at quantity discounts for bulk purchases.
For information, please call 1-800-289-0963.

Contents

Acknowledgments

I would like to thank the following people whose encouragement, insight, and guidance made this book possible: Amberly Finarelli at Andrea Hurst Literary Management for just being the most awesome agent ever; Kate Powers at Adams Media for thinking of me for this project; Chef AJ for her culinary, whole foods, and vegan expertise; Melissa Kay Allen for being my go-to wedding gal; Kirsten Tanner for being my go-to vegan gal; Tiina Kurvi for her careful eye; Jenn Erickson for being a sounding board; and all the vendors and brides I have worked with, who have taught me so much about different cultures, lifestyles, and personalities—you are an inspiration.

Top 10 Simple Ways to Veganize Your Wedding

1. Lead by example and trust in yourself. Don't apologize for your beliefs and your decisions, and others will respect them. If it doesn't feel right . . . don't do it!

2. Practice kindness and giving. Plan with a purpose, give with a cause, and if you do not need anything, suggest donations to charitable vegan organizations.

3. Give your guests the benefit of the doubt. You may be worried (and they may think) that they will miss something with a vegan meal, but serve up a grand offering and chances are no one will care or notice! Make the food the star!

4. Make conscious decisions about your attire. You may be tempted by extravagant silk designer gowns, but you can get a gorgeous gown in vegan-friendly fabric and stun the guests.

5. Get your friends and family on board, and ask that they keep all parties and showers vegan, too!

6. Work with and support like-minded people. Support vegan businesses and local vegan vendors.

7. Gently inform and educate the guests, but do not expect them all to understand or convert. Now is the time for celebration, not for debating issues.

8. Hire a masterful digital photographer to capture your day, and share your photos online with your friends.

9. Treat the animals, the earth, and the guests with kindness, and rejoice in the difference a person can make.

10. Find an amazing vegan baker and show the guests how delectable and decadent vegan cakes, desserts, and pastries can be.

Introduction

EVERY WEDDING IS DIFFERENT. Sometimes the differences are the location, the theme, or the blending of two cultures, and other times they are due to a particular lifestyle that the bride and groom have embraced. In spite of the multitude of possible circumstances, at its core, the basic premise of planning, orchestrating, and pulling off a wedding celebration is virtually the same. It is once you start to add the personal details and nuances of each couple that the wedding takes on a life of its own. As you introduce your vegan lifestyle into the wedding plans, there will definitely be a few twists and turns to your planning, a few more steps to take, feelings to take into consideration, and strong beliefs to respect . . . but it will all be worth it!

As a couple already living a vegan lifestyle, you know what it takes to maintain that lifestyle and live by your beliefs and convictions. Yet, when it comes to wedding planning, you are now involving a whole set of people—vendors, friends, and family—that may or may not be truly familiar with what living a vegan life means. In fact, as the bride and groom, you may even be puzzled how to find the vegan resources you need to plan your wedding or how to even incorporate veganism seamlessly into the wedding plans. So, yes, you may possibly face some challenges as you are planning your wedding, but rest assured there are solutions.

Along the way, questions will arise: How do you let your friends and family know your wedding will be vegan? Do you even have to? How do you include your vegan lifestyle in your wedding planning? How do you find locations and vendors that will be respectful of your choices? How do you introduce the guests to vegan beliefs? How do you blend your beliefs with those of your families? Here is where this book comes in—finally, a resource that covers these topics, and so much more.

As you move through your planning and this book, each chapter contains insights and advice on every aspect of your wedding, from hiring a wedding planner and vendors that share your vision to designing an amazing vegan menu that leaves guests wanting more! This book addresses some of the more common vegan issues you will face as you plan, such as finding a vegan baker or buying that stunning cruelty-free wedding gown, and maybe most importantly, the bride and groom will get advice and tactics for handling some trickier family and guest situations that may arise.

All weddings have their share of challenges, but a vegan wedding may face a few more. You might find your father asking, "Why can't we serve roasted chicken?" Your mother may be swooning over a flowing silk gown, and the guests may be wondering, "What the heck does a vegan wedding mean for me?" Chances are these people would not utter a syllable about your selections if you were planning a soirée incorporating elements of your religion or culture, but throw in veganism, and all bets are off.

When faced with these issues, the vegan couple needs to realize that they are entitled to throw any kind of wedding they want, without apologies. Weddings are about encompassing the interests, personalities, and passion of the bride and groom, and a vegan wedding is no different. Accept these challenges with friendliness and kindness, but also head-on with facts and information the guest can understand. Most of all, give your guests the benefit of the doubt; these are modern ever-changing times and many of them may be right on board with trying a vegan meal and celebrating with you in a vegan-friendly way!

CHAPTER 1

The Vegan Couple

You know the constant commitment it takes to maintain a vegan lifestyle and live by your beliefs and convictions. Now, as you plan your wedding, a whole new set of people—vendors, friends, and family—are involved. Many of these people may not be truly familiar with what living a vegan life means, leaving you with a few extra steps in the planning and the possibility of facing some challenges on this journey. Rest assured, though, your vegan wedding can be beautiful and special without compromising your beliefs.

Preparing for Your Vegan Wedding

Planning any wedding is essentially the same process. It is the incorporation of the nuances of each couple that changes the game plan a little. As a vegan, you have chosen a particular lifestyle that incorporates compassion and ethical treatment of all living things. Of course you are not going to abandon these ideas just because you are getting married, but before jumping into your planning you need to familiarize yourself with some basic wedding-planning preparation first. Once you do that, you can begin to incorporate the vegan ideals into your wedding.

First Things First

The best chance any marriage has of survival is honest and open communication. Hopefully, if you are ready to say "I do," you have had discussions about family and home and values. If not, do it now, before you make one more decision.

You will have plenty of decisions to make as you plan a wedding, but a wedding is a small portion of the life you are hoping to create. As a couple, it is imperative to discuss the issues that will impact your future beyond the wedding day. Discussing these important matters now will ease some of the transition to married couple after the wedding and beyond.

IF YOU ARE BOTH VEGAN:
- Is this a lifestyle you are both committed to for the long haul?
- How would you feel if one of you has a change of heart about veganism?
- Would a change of heart be a "deal breaker"?

IF ONE OF YOU IS NOT A VEGAN:
- Is this a lifestyle the nonvegan is willing to accept and make compromises for? Is the vegan willing to make compromises for the nonvegan? It is a two-way street, folks!
- Will you keep and maintain a completely vegan home? What is the range of wiggle room, if any? For example, leather sofas are out but chicken for dinner for the nonvegan is okay?

- Is the vegan willing to prepare meals for the nonvegan? If so, to what degree—anything but the meat? Or how will it be delegated?
- Will you divide the refrigerator, pantry, utensils, and pots and pans to accommodate both needs?
- When you entertain, will you entertain with vegan menus and values?
- Will you raise your children vegan, vegetarian, or nonvegan?

Get Planning

Once you have some ground rules for the future established, it is time to move on to wedding planning. It is not uncommon to devote as much as a year to planning your big event. This by no means suggests that you must plan for one year, but the longer you give yourself the better chance you will have your pick of vendors and locations, especially if you have your heart set on a specific date.

Some ceremony and reception sites, as well as top vendors, can be booked more than a year in advance. If you are looking to walk the aisle at a vegan locale such as the only organic garden or farm in the area, give yourself plenty of planning time in order to secure the date you want. If you are flexible about the date, you will have a better chance of finding the perfect location and creating the wedding you dream of.

FACT

If you choose to work with only vegan locales and vendors, additional time to plan may be a necessity. While the number of people practicing a vegan lifestyle is growing every day, vegan professionals are not always readily available and accessible in all areas and may be booked far in advance. Give yourself time to plan for the kind of wedding you want.

Questions, Questions, Questions

There is an enormous amount of information available for planning your wedding. The Internet, Facebook, Twitter, magazines, books, bridal shows, not to mention your friends and family—it is much too easy to get caught up in what you should do and what you are supposed to do rather than what you want to do. Together, you and your partner need to devise a set of guidelines and priorities to streamline the planning process.

Begin the planning process by having yourself and your partner answer some very basic wedding-planning questions.

- Will the wedding be strictly vegan? If not, what is/are the compromises?
- What month or season do you want to get married in? Also consider what time of day you want to have your ceremony.
- Would you like to have an indoor or outdoor ceremony? What about the reception?
- Do you need a wedding planner? One who specializes in vegan weddings (or who is knowledgeable in this area) may be helpful, but is it necessary or in your budget?
- Will you only hire vegan vendors?
- Who will officiate your wedding? Do you have a religious leader, a spiritual advisor, or a legal officiant in mind? Will you consider a justice of the peace or another nondenominational officiant?
- What kind of ceremony do you wish to have? Traditional? Spiritual? Religious? Civil? Commitment ceremony?
- What is your budget? Is there wiggle room? Who is paying? This may be the single most important aspect of your planning because it will decide every other area of your wedding.
- How many people will you invite?
- Who will be in your wedding party? Bridesmaids, groomsmen, ushers, flower girl, ring bearer—remember, they aren't necessary, but many people have at least a maid of honor and a best man.
- Do you wish to incorporate a separate theme into your vegan wedding? Recycled retro, nature's beauty, autumn splendor—any idea and theme can be combined and used creatively with a vegan edge.

Diplomacy of Planning

When family dynamics and emotions are involved, it does not take much for tempers to flare and feelings to be hurt, particularly during such an exciting and momentous time. Even in the most congenial families, situations arise. The thought of running off to get married may even cross your mind when your parents, friends, and anyone else who has an opinion starts sharing. No one needs this additional stress. Approach each situation with open communication and consideration, and just maybe the tension can be alleviated or even avoided.

Communication Is the Key to Success

Let's face it: There are some differences that meetings, explanations, and facts are not going to settle. That is just life. If you are lucky, you have a reasonable set of parents, soon-to-be in-laws, and friends who are willing to compromise and communicate in order to keep the planning flowing smoothly. Ultimately, it all comes down to the issues, personalities, and convictions of those involved. And let's be honest, who's paying must be factored in as well.

FACT

Adding what may be an unknown or misunderstood lifestyle to the planning mix may make some family members uncomfortable, causing uneasiness and hostility. Do your best to explain the facts and talk openly about veganism and your beliefs to alleviate this additional stress. Consider inviting everyone to a vegan feast to discuss the plans.

As the bride, you are the major facilitator of all things wedding, but do not hesitate to get your partner involved, especially when it comes to his family. You may want to encourage both mothers to consult with one another on any major events that each is planning. For example, if your mother is hosting your engagement party, your future mother-in-law would probably appreciate feeling like more than an invited guest. She may be more than happy to help out.

Money Is Power

Traditionally, the bride's family plans and finances the majority of the wedding details; however, for a modern wedding it is not uncommon for the financial responsibility to be split amongst all the parties, including the couple. If you're concerned there may be some competition between families, take some steps toward achieving a warm, cooperative environment. Look for aspects of the planning where both sides can be included or opinions solicited. There are other ways to make the groom's family an active part of the wedding.

Watch Out for Your "Friends"

If you think your families have opinions, wait until your friends get involved. If you get lucky, your friends will be mature and understanding enough to be supportive in your plans and decisions and know when to keep their opinions to themselves. But there is almost always someone who feels she needs to voice her opinion—about why she cannot wear a silk dress or leather shoes or why the salad cannot have goat cheese.

Your Wedding, Your Beliefs

You embrace the vegan lifestyle you have chosen every day. You honor and believe in what you feel is right and ethical. Now it is time for you to get married. That means combining families and friends and explaining your lifestyle to some of these people. Some friends and family members may be eager to learn about your veganism; others may not. Either way, have the information readily available to share should the situation arise. Most of all, remember it is your wedding, your beliefs, and you need to be comfortable with your decisions.

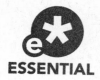

ESSENTIAL

Once you have some basic planning necessities under control and have acquainted yourself with the politics of planning, it is time to start thinking about the "veganization" of your wedding planning. With a solid plan, the addition of vegan ideas and elements will fall into place right alongside the general planning necessities.

Finding Balance

When you chose to live a vegan life it was because you had strong feelings and beliefs about the treatment of all living things, your health, and the well being of the environment. While you may be passionate about this, you must realize there are many who are not, and some of them may be coming to your wedding. As you begin your planning, you and your fiancé need to determine how you are going to handle this issue and what kind of balance, if any, you are willing to strike with the nonvegan guests.

You know veganism encompasses an entire lifestyle of abstaining from any animal products or by-products. However, is this the position you are going to take or even overtly promote at your wedding? Are you going to provide the guests with a complete vegan experience from head to tummy, or will you make concessions here and there to keep your families or the guests happy, even if it means going against what you hold dear? You have to decide how passionately you feel about different issues, what you can live with, and what will keep you up at night.

Explain Your Beliefs

Expect to hear some groans, disbelief, and even puzzlement from some family members and guests when they hear you are throwing a vegan wedding. It is common for people to react this way when they are faced with an unknown, but do not take it personally. Chances are good that this is all based on a lack of knowledge and understanding of what veganism really means.

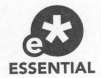

Once you have some basic planning necessities under control and have acquainted yourself with the politics of planning, it is time to start thinking about the "veganization" of your wedding planning. With a solid plan, the addition of vegan ideas and elements will fall into place right alongside the general planning necessities.

Introducing Veganism to the Nonvegan

For many who have never explored the idea of veganism, there are many misconceptions of what being vegan means. Realistically, you have to know there are some out there who cannot grasp the concept of veganism. You can bet that even in the most understanding circles, there is someone who thinks they will be eating nuts for dinner or that you are just plain crazy for not eating meat.

You are under no obligation to tell the guests that you are throwing a vegan wedding. Whether you choose to or not is totally up to you. Many do so that guests will have an understanding of the choices being made, and so they can truly be a part of the wedding with proper vegan-friendly attire, appropriate gifts, etc. When all is said and done, some guests will simply accept the wedding for what it is—a wedding; others will expect nothing less than a vegan wedding; and others may not even notice a difference from any other wedding.

DECIDE WHICH ROUTE YOU WANT TO TAKE AND CONSIDER THE FOLLOWING:

- Send out a note with the Save the Date or start/include information on veganism on your wedding blog/wedding website. Explain what it means to be a vegan and include some vegan resources. Keep the information factual and mainstream. Information is essential to understanding some of the nuances that will take place due to your beliefs.
- Determine how much of the vegan lifestyle you are going to incorporate into your planning. For example, will you ask guests not to wear leather or silk or wool? Or will you be happy with planning from a

vegan perspective and as a couple abide by these "rules," but not expect your guests to?

- Talk openly and honestly about why you chose to be vegan if anyone asks. Arm your wedding party and parents with some basic information (if they are not vegan) so that when Aunt Martha asks, "Why would anyone have a vegan wedding?" they may assist in introducing the idea of veganism to the guests.

Compromises

How do you keep everyone happy and not compromise your own beliefs? It may be a challenge depending on your guests. The younger set and forward thinkers will most likely jump on board without an issue. But your great uncle who grew up on meat and potatoes may not get it no matter what you say.

Bride Versus Groom

Yes, vegans marry other vegans . . . but sometimes vegans fall in love with vegetarians and sometimes even with carnivores! Of course, everything would be simpler if both the bride and groom had similar ideals, but what if they don't? What if a vegan marries an almost-vegetarian, the majority of the guests are not vegan, and the father of the bride (who is footing the entire bill) *loves* his beef? That may be extreme, but don't smirk—it has been known to happen!

Keeping the Family Happy

To you, all of this vegan planning may be simple, but what are you going to do when Dad, who is paying for a portion of the wedding, requests that some meat be served at the reception? What if Mom wants to wear a silk dress? How are you going to keep them happy and not compromise your own beliefs?

Sometimes, parents feel as though the guests will think they are being cheap or the wedding will be less grand or formal if it is vegan. Address these issues by presenting your family with viable vegan options and facts. Explain to your family why this is so important to you and how much it would mean for them to respect your decisions and support you. Show them examples of vegan weddings online and the ideas you have gathered to strengthen your position. A vegan wedding can be every bit as formal and the meal every bit as delicious as any other wedding. If all else fails, ask yourself if you are willing to pay for the wedding yourself if your parents refuse to accept the idea of a vegan wedding.

Know When to Hold 'Em

When some parties, especially the bride or groom, are not vegans, there are choices to be made and compromises to consider. The points below are by no means the only ones you may be confronted with, but they may be some of the most important, and you and your fiancé need to decide where your boundaries are.

- Are you both committed to an entirely vegan wedding?
- Will you consider including some organic cheeses for hors d'oeuvres?
- If the groom is a meat eater, will you consider serving an organic animal protein with the meal? (It is his wedding too!)
- (If you are both vegan) Are you willing to serve organic meat or dairy at your wedding to appease your father who is paying for the majority of the wedding?
- Are you willing to serving a vegetarian menu that includes some organic dairy elements?
- Will you provide different meals for different guests? For example, vegan meals for the vegans and a "traditional" menu for the remainder of the guests?
- Can you block out the minor complaints and criticisms you may hear about the lack of animal protein on your wedding menu? It is rude, but it may happen.
- Are you willing to hire nonvegan vendors if they agree to adhere to your vegan ideals for the wedding day?
- Will you ask your guests to go vegan, including their choice of dress for the wedding?
- Will you ask your bridesmaids to throw a completely vegan bridal shower?

Guests' Participation

There will be some guests who just simply want to buy a gift, show up, and watch you exchange vows. They don't care if the wedding is vegan or if it is on Mars, they are just there for the wedding . . . and maybe a free glass of wine! They have no desire or reason to explore any vegan aspects of the wedding, and may not even realize it is a vegan wedding. Of course, there may be a guest or two or ten that balk at the idea of a vegan wedding, and there is nothing you can do about that. You have to be willing to accept this as well.

On the bright side, you may have friends and family who are open to learning about and embracing veganism—even if just for a day—out of respect for you. If this is the case, you should embrace and celebrate their enthusiasm, too. Be prepared with ideas and information for them. Celebrate their eagerness and willingness to support you.

TRY A FEW OF THESE OPTIONS TO HELP YOUR GUESTS UNDER-STAND AND GET THE RIGHT INFORMATION:

- Supply the guests with a list of items that vegans abstain from. For example, they may know not to wear leather, but not wearing silk or wool never crossed their minds.
- Supply the guests with a list of online or local shops and merchants where they can find vegan-friendly clothing.
- Offer up some menu suggestions or referrals to local restaurants that cater to vegans—they just may want to try out some great vegan food.

Vegan-Friendly Ideas

What's the trick to vegan wedding-planning success, you might ask? First, remember that wedding planning is wedding planning; the same basic steps apply. Once you understand this, begin adding in your vegan ideas and values. Start with what you know. Many of the vegan resources you currently use on a daily basis may have referrals to other vegan services and products you will want to incorporate into your wedding.

Everyone Has to Start Somewhere

You may need to be creative to accommodate your vegan needs and desires. Of course, in certain geographical areas it will be easier than in others. Ask the following people for advice along the way:

- Ask your favorite restaurant if they cater or know of a professional vegan caterer. Inquire about their dessert options, too.
- Vegan restaurants you frequent may even be great venues for the wedding itself.
- Ask the local florist if she has a referral to vegan and/or organic flowers, or if she is willing to use only organically grown flowers for your wedding.
- Shop local vegan vendors and look for eco-conscious and fair-trade products, as well.
- Scour the web for online shops and handmade items. You will be amazed at the beauty and reach of vegan products available for you and your wedding with a few key strokes.

Shop the Web for Vegan-Friendly Solutions

Just about anything and everything can be found on the Internet these days—it has become a vast resource for communication, entertainment, education, and shopping. If you can't find what you need at local stores, you can find it online. You can search for the perfect location for your ceremony and reception or scout out a site for your great green honeymoon.

ALERT

When you purchase from online retailers, select ground delivery instead of air whenever possible. Airplanes have a much greater effect on global warming than vehicles. When you compare products, if all things are equal—product, price, and quality—always choose the retailer that is closest to you. It saves on shipping costs and cuts down on carbon emissions.

To purchase and find the vegan items you desire or want for your wedding, you may have no choice but to turn to the Internet. Not every town or city has a vast selection of vegan resources, but those amazing online shops do! Sites like Etsy host an enormous amount of small businesses that cater to the vegan, more than most could hope to find in their own city.

The web is full of information that can help you plan your vegan wedding; from informational sites to online retailers and vendors, you are sure to find what you are looking for. Searching the Internet can save you a lot of time, and you have the advantage of being able to plan your wedding without changing out of your pajamas.

Green and Vegan—A Perfect Match!

Going green and being a vegan have a lot in common. From saving water resources to soil erosion to the conservation of our land, there is a respect for the environment and a concern for the planet and all things that live and thrive here. Just because you are vegan does not necessarily mean that you are green—and vice versa—but that does not mean you cannot borrow some great green ideas to get your wedding plans moving in the right direction.

Buying the Right Products

Some people think that buying vegan or green products and using these types of services costs more than using "regular" products and services. It doesn't necessarily have to. While sometimes the initial expense may be more, you will save money and the Earth, and stay true to your beliefs by doing so. For instance, the durability of hemp and bamboo fabrics means that they will last longer than their synthetic counterparts. Products made from these fabrics may cost more, but they last much longer and will not wear out and need to be replaced as quickly. Just think, the bridesmaids can keep their dresses for a very long time!

When it comes to planning your vegan wedding, there are many eco-options that will not hurt your pocketbook.

- The average cost of a wedding dress is around $1,300, and it is not uncommon for a bride to pay upward of $3,000 for a designer gown. Bridal gowns made from sustainable, organic, and cruelty-free fabrics can be as much as $1,000 (or more), but generally cost much, much less. You'll pay a fraction of the original price for a used gown, and an heirloom or borrowed gown will be free, except for cleaning costs and possible alteration fees.
- Hemp suits cost about the same as renting a designer-brand tuxedo, but you'll have the added advantage of being able to wear it over and over again.
- If you embrace the concept of reusing, you'll buy things that will serve double duty; they can be used at your wedding then reused in your home. Glassware, dinnerware, table linens, baskets, potted plants, and trees are all items you can incorporate into your postwedding life.

Go Green/Save Green

Shop at local antique shops, thrift stores, and yard sales instead of at bridal boutiques, wedding supercenters, and mass merchandisers to save cash. You'll spend much less, find quality items that can be reused, and enjoy the treasure hunt.

ALERT

If you choose to treasure hunt for items, be aware that not all items will have labels or tags, and sometimes the difference between materials is not distinguishable. You will need to be extra careful about anything you purchase to ensure you are buying cruelty-free items.

THERE ARE OTHER WAYS TO GO VEGAN AND GREEN:
- Make responsible choices when choosing outdoor locations. Choose parks and organic gardens that are set up to be natural yet still accessible to people. A true wilderness location is not equipped to handle human parties. You may do more harm than good by having your wedding in a truly wild setting.

- Be sensitive in the materials you choose. Skip the balloons, crepe paper, and tulle decorations. None are natural and they all just get thrown away.
- Say no to disposables and plastic utensils. Choose items that can be reused or recycled.
- Forgo the disposable cameras. Ask everyone to bring their digital cameras, and guests can e-mail you the photos, put the photos on a disc for you, or share the photos at online sites.
- Think outside the wedding mindset. Purchase items you can reuse, such as a great pair of shoes. Buy something you'll use again, not just something you'll use exclusively for your wedding day.
- Rent or borrow whatever possible. This reduces the need for new items to be made and purchased and greatly slashes your expenses. Items that can be rented or borrowed include altars, trellises, gazeboes, tables and chairs, and other things such as tuxedos, table linens, dinnerware and table settings, glass bowls or vases for centerpieces, and even jewelry and other accessories.
- When it comes to clothing and linens, consider how they will be cleaned. Find a green dry cleaner for your wedding dress, and research tuxedo and table linen rental companies that use green dry cleaning processes.
- Ask yourselves, "Do we really need this?" Cut out all the unnecessary stuff and you'll save money while you help save the environment.

CHAPTER 2

Planning 101—
With a Vegan Twist

Planning a vegan wedding is the same as planning a tradi-tional wedding. It will be exciting, fun, tiring, trying, time consuming, and completely worth it. Now that you have become acquainted with some of the special consider-ations you need to take as you plan a vegan wedding, it is time to get moving and get this wedding planned! Take it all in stride, and the planning will culminate in a beautiful day filled with love and hope for the future.

Where to Start

You already had a life, right? A job, a family, and social obligations, but now you have a wedding to plan on top of all that. Even if you are entertaining the idea of hiring a wedding planner, you still need to be organized, resourceful, and motivated to get this wedding planned. Along the way you will face challenges, make numerous decisions, spend a lot of cash, and still manage to go to work every day!

Get and Stay Organized

You want to enjoy your planning and not forget a thing, right? You not only have a wedding to plan, but the special addition of vegan touches and aspects to incorporate into the plans. It can be a lot to manage, but if you take a few steps to get and stay organized, you can stay on top of the planning and on the right track for success. Keeping the paperwork, swatches, and forms organized will help you keep your sanity from the beginning of the planning until your walk down the aisle.

FACT

Go green with your planning. You can manage most of your wedding planning online and with your tablet, smartphone, or laptop. Vendor communications and great ideas can all be stored online and paper free! Also consider using an online resource like Pinterest to manage all those fabulous decorating ideas!

First, establish a filing system for hard copies of contracts and other forms. Keep them there for safekeeping. For your mobile planning, a three-ring binder with sheet protectors is the way to go. Make copies of contracts for the binder, place swatches and color chips in the pockets, and fill it up with tear outs from magazines and other items that inspire you for your wedding. This system is easy to update, and makes a perfect traveling companion.

Don't Start Planning Until . . .

Where do you begin your planning? Too often the bride takes over as captain of the ship, and the groom is left behind wondering if his opinion matters at all. So, sit down together, just the two of you, and figure out a game plan.

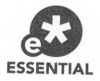

ESSENTIAL

Start your preliminary guest list early. Determine who must be invited (family, closest friends, your boss) and who you would like to invite (distant relatives, long-distance friends, coworkers). It will put your guest list and budget in perspective.

There are two decisions that need to be made right away, as they go hand in hand: guest list and budget. Guests equal money, as the largest portion of your budget goes to the reception and catering. With this in mind, you must first get a preliminary guest list started. What you may think is only 100 invitees could really end up being 200 when it's on paper. Second, you need to have a basic idea of what you have to spend, which can determine how many guests you will ultimately be able to invite. The funds don't need to be completely budgeted out yet, but you do need a working figure.

Priorities

You may think your dress is the most important part of the wedding, but your fiancé may think the music is. How do you come together and move forward? All aspects of wedding planning need to be put in perspective and prioritized. Each of you should write a list of your own top ten wedding priorities. Then compare lists and make one list based on the mutual agreement of both of your wants. This will not only help you understand each other, it will assist greatly when it comes to making budget decisions.

The Wedding Date

At first sight of an engagement ring on your finger, the questions will start coming. While the first thing you're likely to hear is "Congratulations!" it is closely followed by "When's the date?" You won't be able to forge ahead with your other planning until you set a date, as it is the essential element in all your wedding planning. When will you need the ceremony and reception sites? How long do you have to find a dress? When will you require the services of paid professionals such as caterers, photographers, and musicians? These and many other questions will remain unanswered until you've set a date.

Determining Factors

In the preliminary search for a wedding date, be flexible, opting to work with a season or month rather than one particular date. Then look at your schedules and surroundings. Is a particular time of the year busy at work? Is summertime in your city just too hot to have an outdoor wedding? These are all very real circumstances that can affect your decision. Once you examine the pros and cons of these factors as well as the answers to the following questions, possible dates will fall into place.

Making the Decision

Examine some of the major determining factors in selecting a wedding date. A quick glance through these points may help you narrow your choices quickly.

- What season do you prefer? Do you want a country garden wedding in the spring? Does the season matter to you at all?
- Is there a time of year that your family or the groom's family finds particularly meaningful?
- How much time do you need to plan the wedding?
- Does the availability of a ceremony and reception site coincide with your desired date? If you have your heart set on a certain venue, keep in mind the venue may already be booked for that particular date.
- Are there conflicts that exist for you, your family, or attendants (such as another wedding, a vacation)?
- Consider the impact holidays, religious celebrations, and community events may have on your wedding.

- Check with the Parks and Recreation Department, Chamber of Commerce, Community Calendar of Events, and the venue to make sure a major event is not scheduled in the same place on the same day.

Information Overload

Weddings are a big business and the amount of information out there can seem overwhelming. Not to mention the fact that you will need to dive into the world of vegan wedding planning. Taking some time to discover and investigate what all the wedding hoopla is about will help you make informed decisions. There are numerous arenas in which to gather information and become acquainted with ideas for vegan weddings. The Internet, magazines, and other brides are all invaluable resources for your wedding planning.

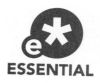

ESSENTIAL

The majority of wedding information you find on the web is not specifically for vegans, but these sites may provide inspiration and ideas you can adapt to fit your vegan wedding. Vegan websites have an enormous amount of general advice, information, and resources. Combine these two resources to steer you toward what you need to know for your wedding.

Hop on the Web

A large portion of your research and preplanning can be done with the computer. There are numerous websites for all aspects of planning, from dresses to the honeymoon. Bridal resources like The Knot, Brides, Junebug Weddings, Wedzilla, and many others are loaded with planning tools, advice, and real wedding photographs as well as paid vendor advertisements. Finding a great resource you like will lead you to others and help your planning progress.

While the majority of wedding resources do not concentrate solely on vegan wedding planning, there is still a good amount of information to be found on these sites. Reading the real-life stories of brides and grooms is eye opening, informative, and inspirational. These sites are great jumping-off points for planning a wedding and finding inspiration that can be translated into your vegan vision.

Hitting the Streets

You can do an enormous amount of research on the Internet, but sometimes you just have to venture out and get up close and personal with vendors and planners and all things wedding.

- **Bridal Shows:** Attending a bridal show may seem like a daunting task, but once you are there, you have so much information at your fingertips. One of the best things about a bridal show is the chance to meet vendors. You can see or taste samples of their work, get a brief idea about their personality or style, and from there decide whether or not to meet with them about your wedding. Wear comfortable shoes, and bring your mom (or a friend), a sturdy bag to tote literature in, and a note pad.
- **Planning Showrooms/Salons:** A huge planning trend is wedding-planning showrooms (sometimes called bridal showrooms or resource centers). At these locations, vendors display their services and you can come at your leisure, with no obligation, to view their work, gather information, and talk to the store personnel about your wedding plans. If there is one in your area, by all means go and take advantage of this great service.

What's Your Wedding Style?

In order to properly plan your wedding, it's imperative that you first decide on the style and formality of the wedding you want. Though you may be eager to get moving on the really fun stuff—interviewing musicians, sampling caterers' cuisine, trying on wedding gowns—figuring out your wedding style first will be time well spent, and will help guide you through the many decisions yet to come.

Defining Your Formality

There are many other factors to consider when determining the level of formality you wish for your wedding. You may also want to take into account some of the following personal factors when determining your wedding's formality.

- **Beliefs:** Do your vegan sensibilities collide with the idea of spending a lot of money and resources on one day? Do you feel that a low-key, eco-conscious, and vegan-centric event represents you well? Or does your veganism not play into your decision on formality at all (i.e., you want what you want!)?
- **Lifestyle:** If you grew up attending grand parties and drinking champagne, will a simple reception at the church hall satisfy you and your guests?
- **Personality:** If you are a super-casual, laid-back gal in your everyday life, would holding a 500-person wedding at the most regal and formal venue make you feel like a princess or like a fish out of water?
- **Locale:** Particular locales conjure up particular feelings and ideas. A country wedding on the farm does not marry well with a ten-foot long train and high heels. The location and the style need to work together.

FACT

Some invitees (including your own family) may have visions of a vegan wedding being too earthy, but a vegan wedding can be anything you want it to be. It can be glamorous, quirky, vintage, country, or traditional, all while staying true to your ideals. Don't get sidetracked by others' mistaken assumptions.

Selecting a Theme

You may be having a vegan wedding, but that does not necessarily need to be the theme of your day. It can be, but it can also just be a regular component of the wedding planning. A theme can definitely make for a unique wedding that stands apart from all others. Depending on the theme, you can explore your fantasies of living in another time or transport your guests to another place. The theme of the wedding should work with your locale and the formality of your wedding, but most importantly, it should reflect your style.

ESSENTIAL

Contrary to popular belief, vegan does not have to be the theme of your wedding. It is a circumstance of your wedding and an underlying commitment, but you can also include a theme or style to complement your personalities.

A wedding does not have to have a theme, and many couples choose to forgo selecting an actual or literal theme altogether. One thing you should also remember is that if you throw a theme wedding, be sure to let the guests in on the plan. Part of the fun is for everyone to be involved. If your theme would be enhanced by the guests dressing the part, be sure to include information on costume shops in the Save the Date or in a separate mailing.

Creative Development

Don't be overwhelmed thinking you have to come up with a theme or some grand design plan for your wedding. You do not need a theme to have a beautiful wedding, nor does your wedding need to be over the top. A beautiful, cohesive look does not require a ton of cash, but it may require some thought. One of the easiest ways to develop a creative element is to carry out a consistent look by incorporating similar elements of design into the reception and ceremony.

A Design Plan

To start designing your wedding, look for inspiration in your everyday life. A favorite vacation destination, a favorite flower, a hobby, the design style of your home, even your favorite color can be an inspiration for your wedding design. You can also look for a design motif that appeals to you (i.e., a natural element such as a hummingbird or flower) and incorporate it into your invitations, programs, and other areas of the wedding.

ESSENTIAL

If you select a monogram as a design aspect of your wedding, do not use the monogram representing your new last name until after the wedding ceremony, when you are officially married. That is, of course, unless you and your fiancé's last names already start with the same letter.

So, just how do you come up with that special detail you want to use? Here are some sources of inspiration:

- Your favorite color or a favorite color of the groom or close family member
- A theme you currently have in your home—shabby chic, vintage, modern, sleek
- A favorite flower
- A favorite vacation destination
- A favorite pastime

- A favorite era (1920s, 1950s, etc.)
- History of the town or location where you are marrying

Tick . . . Tick . . . Tick . . .

Now that you have some of the basics down, you may think you have all the time in the world, but beware: The last thing you want is to suddenly discover that it's three months before your wedding and you don't have a dress yet. A well-planned wedding is all about the schedules. Be aware of some basic time and planning considerations to ease your mind and assist you in getting your top choice in everything from locations to vendors to dresses.

Get on Schedule

Though your tendency may be to procrastinate in the early months, don't! Draw up a schedule, and stick to it. If it can be done months before the wedding, do it months before the wedding. Don't worry—there will be plenty to do as the wedding draws near. Wouldn't you rather be free to be pampered or deal with last-minute details in the weeks prior to the ceremony instead of being bogged down by tasks that could have (and should have) been done much earlier?

Plan to secure the key items in your wedding (ceremony site, reception site, caterer, photographer, flowers, gown, rings, and music) as far in advance as possible. Starting early gives you the breathing room to take your time and make unrushed choices.

CHAPTER 3

Creating the Budget

The B-word—otherwise known as the budget—is the nasty little detail that no one really wants to talk about. Your budget has a very big influence on your wedding. It will dictate the size and style of your wedding as well as other aspects such as flowers, music, photography, video, transportation, and so on. No matter what you have to spend, a wedding is a large investment, and while talking money is not the fun part of the wedding planning, it is a necessary part.

Time to Talk Money

Until you have a frank discussion about money, the wedding budget is the proverbial elephant in the room. As you move through the process of determining your budget, just remember a wedding can be beautiful no matter how much or how little you spend or what type of wedding you are having. As you budget, it is important to remember basic wedding costs are the same—all brides need a dress, yours just happens to be vegan.

The Facts, Like It or Not

Too often, couples sit down to sort out the wedding budget with no sense of what a wedding costs or what it takes to get them from A to Z. They have grand ideas, but no concept of how those ideas translate into reality, or how much those ideas really cost. When it is time to set the budget, it is important to be realistic and to figure out how your wedding is really going to be paid for. Armed with some simple advice and a few pointers, you can get started on mapping out your budget and move on to dresses and flowers and cake tastings.

WHAT YOU NEED TO KNOW TO BUDGET

1. Know who may be contributing monetarily—your groom, your parents, his parents—and honestly discuss expectations and finances.
2. Prioritize the areas of your wedding so you can spend money on what's most important to you.
3. The date you select will affect your final costs. Prime- or high-season wedding dates are considered to be from April through October.
4. Don't ignore your own personal taste. If you have grown up eating at the finest restaurants, a cake and punch reception at the local community center is probably not going to satisfy you, but it might work for someone else.

It'll Cost You!

It is hard to make a blanket statement about what weddings cost. Important factors to consider are the geographic area in which you live or in which you will be marrying. An average wedding in New York City will set you back more than the same type of wedding in Little Rock.

FACT

The single biggest wedding expense you will incur is your reception. As a rule, expect half of your total budget to go toward those costs, which include the menu and the venue. The remainder of the budget is divided amongst the other wedding costs, with percentages varying based on your priorities.

To get a basic idea of local wedding costs, ask recently married friends and check out local wedding websites (many vendors post prices). It would be invaluable for you to call a wedding planner and schedule a budget consultation. Many planners will charge an hourly fee, and you can pick their brains for budget information.

Traditional Expenses

While the bride's parents traditionally financed a major portion of the wedding, it is completely commonplace for the groom's parents to contribute to the budget. As couples marry later in life and have the financial means to do so, the bride and groom have also come to finance a portion, or sometimes the entire wedding, themselves.

As you plan, you may encounter obstacles with parents and other budgetary contributors (if any) for any number of issues, including your vegan ideals. All couples have some issues working out the budget, no matter what style of wedding they are planning. If this is the case, you will have to try and work through the differences with the contributor if you want their help with the budget, decide to make compromises, or choose to pay for the wedding yourself and answer to no one.

Be My Guest

If you're like most brides, compiling your guest list can be challenging . . . unless, of course, you have an open-ended budget and unlimited reception space. Not only do you need to figure out who is going to make the cut, you also need to decide who is going to have a say in the process and, on top of it all, make the list manageable enough to stay within the budget without sacrificing the guest's comfort or your style.

Who to Invite

For the important and possibly delicate task of determining who is invited to the wedding, work with your fiancé and families to create a guest list that suits your wedding plans. If you are like most brides, you will need to make hard decisions, as will your fiancé and your families. So, when it is time to tackle the guest list, follow these simple steps and establish some guidelines to get you moving on the right path.

Dividing the Guest List

In most cases the guest list is divided evenly between the families, regardless of who is paying for what, with the bride's parents, groom's parents, and couple each inviting one-third of the guests. The next step is to list everyone you'd ideally like to have, so you can see if the total number is beyond your reach or not.

Setting Boundaries

If the guest list is too long, establish some boundaries to trim it down to size. Just remember, you must apply all rules across the board. Making exceptions for certain people is the single best way to offend others and create more headaches for yourself. You may want to consider implementing any or all of the following policies:

- **No children:** The fact that you're not inviting children is indicated to parents by the fact that their children's names do not appear anywhere on the invitation. Just to be safe, however, make sure your mother (and anyone else who might be questioned) is aware of your policy. What age you choose as a cut-off point between children and young adults is up to you.
- **No coworkers:** If you were inviting people to the wedding to strengthen business ties, this may not be the best option, but if you do need to

cut somewhere, and you feel comfortable excluding work acquaintances, this may be the way to go.

- **No third-, fourth-, or twice-removeds:** If you have a large immediate family, you may want to exclude distant relatives, with whom you have no regular social interaction.
- **No "and Guest":** While you will certainly want to allow any attached guests to bring their significant others, the same does not necessarily need to extend to unattached guests. Remember, however, that married and engaged guests must always be invited along with their spouses and fiancés. Likewise, each of your attendants should be given the option to bring a guest, even if they're not involved in a relationship.
- **No regrets:** Because it's realistic to anticipate some regrets, it has become popular for couples to have an A-list and a B-list; the Bs receive invites as the As decline the invitation. If you need to make cuts, forgo the B-list invites.

The Vegan Budget

All weddings have similar expenses, and now that you are familiar with those, it is time to get serious about what you can expect when you plan a vegan wedding. It is time to zero in and really concentrate on the special planning needed to make your wedding fabulously vegan, and whether or not that will hurt your pocketbook. You need to understand how your vegan beliefs may impact your budget.

Special Considerations

So, what are the budgetary concerns of a vegan wedding? Will it cost you more to go vegan at your soirée? Could it actually be cost effective? Will it cost less? Is it just a matter of style and preference, as with all weddings? The answer is all of the above.

Generally, you can expect the following budget issues when planning a vegan wedding.

- **Meals and Menu:** Generally, vegetarian and vegan meals will cost less than a meal with an animal protein. However, if you choose to go semivegan and offer some dairy, or even an organic/grass-fed animal protein, your costs may go up due to the multiple options and extra preparation and service staff required.
- **Organic Options:** Organic is good for the Earth and it is good for people, but not all caterers and florists are using organic products. If this is your desire for food and florals, you must specify this and be sure that the vendor can deliver on his organic promises, and at what cost.
- **Planner:** Do you need a vegan wedding planner? Will a vegan wedding-planning specialist cost more? Maybe; maybe not. Specialists in their field can often command a higher price, and a wedding planner who will need to spend extra hours researching vegan ideas and ideals will most likely pass along the cost to you.
- **Cakes and Pastries:** Vegan bakers have been around for a long time, but good vegan bakers may come at a price. Often, you can get a "regular" wedding cake for a song. In fact, some locales even include it in their plans, but when you go with a vegan cake or dessert, the cost may be higher. That is changing as vegan bakers become more mainstream and accessible.
- **The Dress:** Typically, sustainable, cruelty-free fabrics, and even man-made fabrics, will cost less than the fine silks and silk blends many designers use.

Of course these are not the only expenses you need to keep an eye on, just a few of the major aspects of planning that can really impact your spending power.

ALERT

If you ask for any customization on the menu, be sure to get it in writing and have any additional costs detailed. This includes the concessions and arrangements made for vegetarian or vegan ingredients as well as the inclusion of organic ingredients.

What Kind of Wedding?

Of course your wedding will be vegan, but what else will it be? First on the agenda, decide on the type of wedding you want. Your job is to try to construct a budget based on your desires, using the resources available. Perhaps you and your fiancé don't even want a big, formal (or semiformal) wedding. You may both shy away from frills and thrills, preferring to avoid much of the headache and expense by holding a small, simple affair. If this is how you want to go, there are plenty of options: a backyard wedding, a wedding in a home, a civil ceremony—it's up to the two of you. Or you may decide that you want the grand, traditional wedding. In either case, planning expenses becomes particularly important. You'll want to make every dollar go as far as it possibly can.

The Wedding Fund

After you decide on the type of wedding you'd like to have, you'll need to figure out exactly how you're going to afford it. The amounts you allocate yourself will help you determine the number of guests you can invite, the location of your reception, the food you will serve, the number of photographs you will have taken, the flowers on display, and just about every other element of the celebration.

ESSENTIAL

Some (nonvegan) caterers or locales may charge an additional fee for going vegan if it is out of their normal service range (for example, if they must restock their condiments and pantry with vegan items for your wedding). Requesting all organic ingredients may also drive up your final cost.

There are two ways of going about setting a budget. The first is to determine the amount of money that's available right now. This will include any money you and your fiancé may have squirreled away for the event as well as any contributions that you're aware of. For instance, you might know exactly how much your parents have saved in your wedding fund. The total of these resources is your total budget—assuming that you're planning on paying cash for the bulk of your wedding expenses.

If there's no wedding fund but you're pretty sure your parents will want to chip in and help defray the cost of the whole shindig, try tallying up the cost of your ideal wedding before asking for financial assistance. You may find that you'll get a better response if you have a ballpark figure to present rather than asking for a vague contribution.

Cut Here to Spend There

As you plan, there will be certain items, certain vendors, that you will fall in love with. Sadly, a few may be out of your monetary reach. Stepping out of your budgetary bounds is not wise, but if you can find a way here and there to scale back on other aspects, you just might be able to get that designer gown or celebrity photographer.

Can You Spare a Discount?

Talented and respectable vendors may offer slight discounts for off nights (Thursdays), last-minute bookings, and weddings in off-season months like January, but for the most part, you are not going to be able to talk them into shaving thousands of dollars off their price. Most vendors are usually willing to negotiate with their packages, exchanging one thing for another, for example; it doesn't hurt to ask the photographer to swap a large framed engagement photo for some extra pages in your wedding album.

Quick Cost Cutters

Vegan or not, there are some ways to cut some of that fluff out of the budget to make room for those extra necessities.

- Have fewer attendants. This means fewer bouquets, boutonnières, and thank-you gifts.
- Skip the favors.
- Consider a weekday, Friday evening, or Sunday to defray costs. Saturday is the most popular and, therefore, the most expensive time for a wedding.

- Don't plan for a meal-time reception. An afternoon event (between lunch and dinner) or an adult cocktail party is a great option, and you can offer hors d'oeuvres and cake rather than a full meal.
- Have a friend ordained to marry you.
- Consider décor options other than floral arrangements. Use lanterns and soy or flameless candles (if they are allowed), or potted plants.
- Skip the champagne and have the guests toast with whatever they are drinking.
- Trim one hour off the reception time. Many venues book weddings in five-hour time blocks, but depending on your event, three to four hours may be plenty of time. You will save on drinks and musician/DJ time.
- Downsize the wedding cake and order sheet cake to be cut and served from the back.

Hey, Big Tipper

Brides and grooms often overlook one very substantial expense—tips! Depending upon the size of your reception, tipping can easily add a few hundred to a few thousand extra dollars to your costs. Some wedding professionals include a gratuity in their contract then expect an additional tip at the reception. As a result, whom to tip and how much can often be a perplexing dilemma.

Why Tip?

By the time the wedding day rolls around, you will have already paid these vendors a lot of money. Many couples often forget, or simply overlook, this last potential budget buster. So, do you really need to tip vendors? The real answer is maybe. Tipping is and should continue to be a reward for extraordinary service. The scale of your wedding, your wedding venue, and your geographical location will influence final tipping amounts. On a final note, if you cannot afford to tip everyone, a glowing thank-you card is always appreciated.

Wedding Budget Worksheet

Item	Projected Cost*	Deposit Paid	Balance Due	Who Pays?

Wedding Consultant

Fee				
Tip (usually 15–20%)				

Pre-wedding Parties

Engagement**				
Site rental				
Equipment rental				
Invitations				
Food				
Beverages				
Decorations				
Flowers				
Party favors				
Bridesmaids' party/luncheon				
Rehearsal dinner**				
Site rental				
Equipment rental				
Invitations				
Food				
Beverages				
Decorations				
Flowers				
Party favors				
Weekend wedding parties				

*(including tax, if applicable) **(if hosted by bride and groom)

CHAPTER 4

The Support System

With your engagement comes excitement, not just for you, but also for those closest to you. Involving your nearest and dearest in the festivities as members of the wedding party is an honor. Whether it's your best friend, your future sister-in-law, your little sister, or even your mother, these people have signed on to stick with you through the delights and frustrations of wedding planning.

The Selection Process

Choosing a wedding party from your many friends and family members can be quite difficult. Add to that the obligation of long-ago promises and family wishes, and the task can be even more complicated. What every bride needs to remember when making these decisions is to surround herself with supportive, loving people who will contribute to making this a special time in her life.

ALERT

Being part of a wedding is a big and often expensive responsibility. You want to give everyone ample time to plan and save. Six months is the absolute minimum amount of notice you need to give everyone involved.

How Many? And Who?

Your wedding party can be as big or as small as you like. Formal weddings usually have a larger number of attendants than informal ones, but you can bend tradition if you think it's appropriate. Think about which of your close friends and family members you and your groom would really like to have in the wedding. Brides often feel obligated to have certain people in the wedding, even if they're not that close. But surrounding yourself with close friends and family members you can depend on may lead you to discover those prewedding parties, fittings, and rehearsals are going more smoothly than you expected—and are even fun!

ESSENTIAL

Don't bow to your mother's pressure to include your cousin as a bridesmaid if you really don't like her. However, if not asking her promises to cause family strife, you may want to consider including the cousin in some other way—asking her to do a reading, for example.

Traditionally, there are an equal number of bridesmaids and ushers, but there is no reason why you have to adhere to this. The general guideline is one usher for every fifty guests. One concern is that all the bridesmaids have a partner to walk them down the aisle and dance with them during scheduled dances at the reception. But having a couple of extra ushers is no crime. They can walk with each other down the aisle, and they probably won't shed a tear over not dancing in the traditional wedding party dance at the reception.

Special Circumstances

A wedding party is no longer about lining up the girls on one side and the boys on the other. There really are no strict rules as long as good judgment is used. This is the twenty-first century, and bridal parties have finally entered it. The "new" wedding party is about including those closest to you, those who are supportive and accepting and happy to be a part of your special day, whoever they may be. Special circumstances may arise, and here is how to handle the most common.

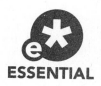

ESSENTIAL

If you're having a hard time deciding between two women for the role of your honor attendant, dual titles may make your life easier. If you have two sisters, for example, and one of them is married and one isn't, voilà! You have a maid of honor and a matron of honor. Divide the duties equally between them.

Distant Maid of Honor

Should distance stop you from having your best friend beside you on your special day? The maid of honor has considerable responsibility before the wedding. You should keep in mind that an out-of-town maid of honor can't be expected to help you with as much of the prewedding planning as someone who lives locally. Just establish as early as possible what it is you would like her to do from afar. Spell out your expectations for her so she knows how she can be helpful even without being in the same time zone.

Maid or Matron or Mommy?

The word "maid" suggests a single woman, but there's nothing wrong with having married attendants. They're still called bridesmaids, but a married maid of honor is called a matron of honor. Even if you have pregnant bridesmaids, many designers now offer maternity-style bridesmaid dresses. Bear in mind that if any of your attendants (particularly the maid or matron of honor) will be eight-and-a-half-months pregnant at the time of your wedding, you may need a standby.

All Mixed Up!

What if your best friend is a guy? There's no reason why he shouldn't be included in your wedding party. Just don't make him wear a dress, dance with an usher, or do any of the traditionally "feminine" duties, such as helping you get into your wedding gown or arranging your train and veil. If he's taking the place of your maid of honor, he's called the honor attendant; if not, he's simply another attendant. He stands at your side, and in the processional and recessional he can walk in before the rest of the bride's attendants. Or, if there are more bridesmaids than ushers, he can escort one of the bridesmaids.

It's also perfectly acceptable to have a female usher (or two) at your wedding, providing the female in question is comfortable with the idea. While she certainly doesn't have to wear a tux and she shouldn't wear a bridesmaid's dress, she should wear something that coordinates with the rest of the wedding party.

Attendants' Duties

While you may be counting on help from the wedding party, oftentimes the bridesmaids and groomsmen aren't sure what they're supposed to do before or at the wedding. At one time, the bridesmaids' main functions were to guard the bride from evil spirits and bear witness that she was not being forced into marriage against her will; the best man was charged with the task of keeping potential abductors from absconding with the bride prior to the wedding day. But that was then, this is now, and the attendants have a much more modern set of duties to attend to.

Maid/Matron of Honor

The maid of honor (or matron of honor) is the bride's legal witness and personal assistant throughout the wedding process. Her more specific duties include:

- Helps the bride with addressing envelopes, and recording wedding gifts
- Arranges/Hosts a bridal shower
- Assists with shopping and other prewedding tasks
- Collects funds and organizes group gift to the bride
- Brings the groom's ring to the ceremony and holds it until the ring exchange
- Signs the marriage certificate as a witness
- Stands in the receiving line (optional)
- Makes sure the bride looks perfect for all the pictures
- Dances with the best man during the attendants' dance at the reception
- Participates in the bouquet toss if single
- Helps the bride change into getaway clothes

Best Man

The best man is the groom's right-hand man. He assists him in getting ready, helps calm nerves, and basically acts as the go-to guy on the wedding day. Additionally, he organizes the bachelor party. He pays for his own formalwear, drives the groom to the ceremony, and holds the bride's ring until it's needed during the ceremony.

The best man is also charged with handing over the checks to the officiant just before or after the ceremony. He may also be asked to take care of paying other service providers, such as the chauffeur or the reception coordinator. If this is to be part of his duties, your groom (or the groom's family) will give the best man the payments ahead of time, which he'll then pass on to the appropriate parties.

Bridesmaids and Ushers

You're asking a lot of the girls who become your bridesmaids, so make sure they're up to the task. At a minimum, they should be ready and willing to help with the following:

- Assist the bride and maid of honor with prewedding errands and activities
- Help organize and run the bridal shower
- Keep a record of the gifts you receive at the shower and who gave what
- Assist you, in any way, on the wedding day
- Participate in the bouquet toss if single
- Stand in receiving line (optional)

Groomsmen and Ushers

Like the bridesmaids, the groomsmen are an additional support system for the bride and groom. They participate in prewedding festivities and assist the couple on the wedding day. Many times the groomsmen and ushers are one and the same. In larger weddings, additional ushers may be needed to seat the guests. Their duties also include:

- Arrive at the wedding location early to help with setup
- Assist in gathering the wedding party for photographs
- Attend to last-minute tasks such as lighting candles, tying bows on reserved rows of seating, etc.
- Roll out aisle runner immediately before processional
- Direct guests to the reception and hand out preprinted maps and directions to those who need them
- Collect discarded programs and articles from the pews after the ceremony
- Help decorate newlyweds' car (optional)

Kids' Stuff

For some, having children be a part of the wedding is a must; for others, they would prefer to give it no thought at all. Whether you choose to include the little ones in the wedding party is entirely up to you. But, you have to admit, watching the little ones walking the aisle as flower girl and ring bearer is pretty cute.

Etiquette does not dictate that you must have a flower girl or ring bearer at your wedding. These roles are there for the purpose of incorporating children in your ceremony. In general, it's young family members who are chosen as flower girl or ring bearer (the distinction is no longer gender specific). The flower child walks down the aisle ahead of the bride and scatters flower petals at her feet. The ring bearer carries a velvet cushion or silver tray on which the (stand-in) wedding bands are held until needed.

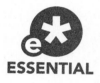

ESSENTIAL

Little ones can be unpredictable, especially those under five (but that is by no means the cutoff age for unpredictable behavior). Be prepared for anything and don't let it ruin your day. Just be happy if they make it down the aisle. And never, ever tie the real wedding rings onto the ring bearer's pillow!

For an older child, the role of junior bridesmaid may be in order. Junior bridesmaids are usually between ten and fourteen; flower girls between four and nine. Little boys, usually under ten, can be ring bearers. Other little boys and girls, called trainbearers, can walk behind the bride, carrying her train.

A Little Help from Your Friends

Most brides cannot justify or simply do not want twenty bridesmaids, but many feel there is no other way to involve friends they would like to be a part of their wedding. Well, no worries, there is much to be done, and delegating tasks will ease your workload while allowing others to contribute their talents and skills to your wedding.

What They Can Do

Below are some ideas for including friends and other special people in your wedding and wedding planning.

- Acting as hostess/hostesses on the wedding day, directing guests to their seats, providing necessary information, and assisting with the guestbook and gifts.
- If one has beautiful penmanship, ask if she will assist with invitations and place cards.
- Have them man the gift table at the reception, making sure that gift cards are secured to the gifts, and most importantly, that gifts are secured once the reception begins.
- Try a favor-making party with these friends, where they can assist in making/assembling favors and other small items you need for the wedding.
- Ask them to be a reader at the wedding.
- If they are musically inclined, ask them to play a musical selection or sing a song or two at the wedding or reception.
- If one of your friends is up to the task (and you do not have a wedding planner or just need some additional assistance), ask her to act as a point person on the wedding day, ensuring vendors have arrived, the wedding party has their flowers, the reception is set up appropriately, etc.
- Ask a vegan friend to double check the caterer (if they are not strictly a vegan caterer) to ensure everything is in order (no cream for the coffee, no honey for the tea, and no butter for the bread).

Vegan Ambassador

Chances are pretty good that if you are living the vegan life, you have some vegan friends. Chances are also good that there will be some puzzled guests at the ceremony. Even if you have made it known the wedding is vegan, people do not always pay attention, and there will inevitably be a guest or two wondering when the main course (a.k.a. the meat) is being served. Ask one of your trusty vegan friends to be a vegan ambassador, offering answers and information to any guests who may have questions.

Wedding Planners

Most women today are already leading busy lives juggling a social calendar and a career. Add to that the proposition of planning a wedding, and some women find their stress and anxiety levels rising. Even if you have the time to spare, planning a wedding is not always about having the time to plan, but having the knowledge. An experienced wedding planner can show you the ropes and offer a tremendous amount of guidance when it comes to planning your wedding.

FACT

Hiring a vegan wedding planner is not necessary to ensure the vegan job gets done correctly. Wedding planners are experts in the wedding field, and plan weddings every day with religions and cultures that are different from their own. Of course, if you wish to support vegan vendors, that is a different story.

Types of Wedding Planners

A wedding planner's purpose is not to take over the plans (unless that's what you hire her to do), but rather to assist and guide you through the planning process, offering creative ideas, time-saving techniques, and organizing all of the aspects of the wedding day. To accommodate the range of needs and budgets for today's bride and groom, wedding planners offer an assortment of services. The following descriptions are generalities that should help you understand the basics when planning services.

- **Full-service planning:** The planner works with a couple from the beginning of the planning, but she may be called in at any point during the planning. In brief, the planner can assist with budgeting, finding and selecting venues and vendors, running wedding-related errands, and following up on all of the details. She is the bride's right-hand man and point person from start to finish. A full-service wedding planner may also assist with event design and styling aspects of the wedding.
- **Month of:** A month-of planner may be hired at any time (earlier is better to ensure you get to work with the planner you want), but she typically begins her essential work one to two months prior to the wedding day. The planner offers referrals early in the planning, and then organizes and fine tunes your carefully laid plans as the day draws nearer. She will manage the final wedding details, such as

calling the wedding day vendors and creating an itinerary. She will also be present at the rehearsal and on the wedding day to ensure things are running smoothly and on time.

- **Day of:** This service assumes and expects the bride to plan her wedding, finalize all the details and logistics, and create her own itinerary. The planner will then use the information the bride has provided to direct the rehearsal and guide the couple through the wedding day.
- **Hourly services:** If you feel you could use the services of a wedding planner in some areas but are not interested in hiring someone to be with you on the wedding day, many planners will meet with couples on an hourly basis.

Fees for wedding planners vary: Some charge a flat rate; others ask for 10–20 percent of the total cost of the wedding; and some charge by the hour. A planner's experience, expertise, and the geographical location influence fees. Most planners are willing to customize their services to accommodate your specific needs. Finally, remember a wedding planner is someone you hire that will work for you. While you may be working with a location manager at your venue, this is not your wedding planner.

Does She Understand Veganism?

Wedding planners are used to working with couples from all cultures and with a variety of different lifestyles. With research and a careful ear, an experienced planner can take on just about any wedding and please the couple. But what does this mean to you and your vegan wedding? It means that you can work with any planner of your choosing, whether she be a vegan expert or not, but that she must be willing to research and respect your vegan decisions and enforce them on the wedding day. Typically, you will be able to tell if a planner is sincere when you meet with her.

ALERT

If working with a vegan planner and supporting vegan vendors in general is essential to you, that should be one of the first questions you ask on the phone, prior to scheduling any meeting. No use in wasting anyone's time!

Let's Get Specific

There are basic questions and qualifications you should cover and look for when hiring a wedding planner, but you have specific needs, too. Don't be shy about covering some of these specific points pertaining to vegan weddings while you are on the phone.

- Do you understand what veganism is?
- Have you ever planned a vegan wedding?
- Are you familiar with some or any specific needs a vegan wedding may have?
- If you are not vegan, are you willing to respect our decisions and do the extra research it will take to accomplish our vegan wedding plans?
- Will there be any additional charges for research due to the vegan planning?
- Do you have access to vegan vendors or know where to look for vegan vendors?

Questions to Ask

After establishing some vegan guidelines, it is time to get down to business with the other important aspects you will want to look for in a wedding planner. You want to select someone who listens to your needs and ideas, and who you feel is capable of handling the job. Ask friends, family, and coworkers for referrals. Below is a list of questions that should help you find the right wedding planner.

- How long has the consultant been in business? Many years in business should indicate experience and contacts. It also means that a consultant is probably reputable, as he or she hasn't been run out of town by unhappy clients.
- Is the consultant full time or part time?
- Can you get references from former clients?
- Is the consultant a full-service planner, or does his or her expertise lie only in certain areas?
- If the consultant isn't a full-service planner, what services does he or she handle?

- What organizations is the consultant affiliated with?
- Is the consultant scheduled to work with any other weddings that are on the same day as yours? You don't want your consultant to be too busy with someone else to meet your needs.
- How much or how little of the consultant's time will be devoted to your wedding?
- What is the cost? How is it computed? (Hourly? Percentage? Flat fee?)
- If the consultant works on a percentage basis, how is the final cost determined?
- Exactly what does the quoted fee include (or omit)?

Vendors That Share Your Vision

There are plenty of wedding professionals out there ready and waiting for your phone call or e-mail, but are they all ready and willing to accept the task of working with you and understanding your vegan wedding? A vendor does not necessarily need to be a vegan or specialize in vegan weddings to get the job done for you, but she should respect your decisions and be committed to carrying out those ideals and wishes on the wedding day.

Working with the Pros

After all of the time you have spent carefully planning, on the wedding day, these carefully laid plans are in the hands of your vendors. The vendors you hire and the relationships you establish with them play a major role in the success of the wedding day. When trying to staff your wedding production, if you look in the right places, you will find qualified, reliable vendors that meet your needs.

ESSENTIAL

If you cannot find vegan specialists, most vendors, if skilled in their craft, are capable of working with couples on any type of wedding, no matter the theme, culture, or other special circumstances. Look for professionals that will protect your vegan beliefs, be eco-responsible, and are socially ethical in their lives and business practices.

Finding the Right Ones

Vendors, if chosen wisely, are your greatest wedding day allies. Professional and reliable vendors are available in all areas and for all budgets and specialties. Researching their qualifications and making sure you and the vendor have a good rapport in the personality and style departments are important steps in ensuring wedding day success. You can begin your search for wedding vendors in the following places:

- **The Internet:** From major, national websites, you can find links to local professionals. You can also explore the websites of professional wedding organizations for referrals to their members. Don't forget to check out local websites and bridal blogs.
- **Regional bridal publications:** This is where to find the professionals and local happenings in a particular region. They also have advertisements for vendors in most categories.
- **Bridal shows:** Want to meet some vendors face to face? Here you can see samples of their work and get an overall impression of their style and demeanor to determine whether or not you would like to meet with them later to discuss their services or get more information.
- **Referrals:** Friends and family members are a great source for leads on vendors. If you know someone whose judgment you trust, relying on their feedback about a vendor is particularly helpful.
- **Vendors, venues, wedding planners:** Referrals from qualified professionals you have hired or trust are definitely worth looking into.
- **Everyday life:** Many of the vegan shops and businesses you frequent may have a wealth of resources for your wedding.

Help Wanted: Vegan Vendors

Along with the above key factors for finding vendors, you may want to pursue finding vegan vendors. Depending on the area you live in or are marrying in, this may prove to be easy or very difficult. While veganism is becoming more mainstream, wedding professionals who specialize in vegan weddings are not necessarily accessible in all areas of the country.

You do have options! First, consult any local vegan establishments for recommendations (chances are you already know these hot spots in your area). Next, look into vegetarian and vegan associations, societies, and local groups. Finally, if those options do not provide enough of a pool to select from, look into green vendors. They may lead you in the right direction.

Signing on the Dotted Line

When hiring vendors, you should interview each one thoroughly. Search the Internet for reviews about the vendor—unhappy brides tend to find a way to make themselves heard. Also, ask each vendor for references; but clearly, a vendor is not going to give you the phone numbers of people who are unhappy with their services. Finally, keep in mind that advertisements are placed by the vendors themselves, so they are going to be glowing endorsements. Once you find the professionals you are happy with, be sure to get a written contract with each one.

CONTRACT CHECKLIST
- ○ Date of the event
- ○ Time of the event
- ○ Arrival/Setup time of the vendor
- ○ Name of the company
- ○ Name of the person/persons performing the service (if applicable)
- ○ Attire/Dress code (if applicable)
- ○ Location/Locations of the event
- ○ Detailed description, including the type and scope of services to be performed
- ○ Any specialized or extra services or provisions discussed, such as vegan considerations/supplies/requests
- ○ Deposit information: how much and when it is due
- ○ Payment information: how much and due dates
- ○ Cancellation policies
- ○ Signatures of both parties

CHAPTER 5

Location, Location, Location

The location of your ceremony and reception may be one of the most important aspects of your entire wedding. You want it to be someplace special, beautiful, and meaningful. The locale is part of the personality of the event and the main backdrop for this amazing wedding you have created. Finding just the right place does take time, but it will be worth it. Luckily for you, the options are endless, from traditional choices such as your place of worship to saying "I do" at an organic vineyard, you can make your wedding one of a kind.

The Perfect Place

It used to be easy—a wedding ceremony was held at the family church followed by a reception at the local hotel or in the church's community room. That was then, this is now. Today, a marriage is a marriage, but a wedding is another thing entirely. Consequently, the choice of a wedding venue, both for the ceremony and reception, is one of the most important elements of your wedding. It sets the tone for the planning and plays a major role in all stylistic decisions.

Start Looking Now

The first thing you have to do is find a venue. Some will tell you to set the ceremony date first and then find a reception site. Many couples, however, try to do just the opposite. Of course, this is like the chicken-and-the-egg question. What it really comes down to is whether you are more particular about the site of the wedding ceremony or the reception.

If you just have to be married in the church where you grew up, and its available dates don't coincide with the dates available at the reception site you're considering, then you'll just have to find another banquet hall. On the other hand, if you want your reception in a certain location but the location of the actual ceremony doesn't really matter to you (you'll even consider a civil ceremony on the premises), your choice is obvious.

ESSENTIAL

During the peak wedding months of April through October, competition for wedding sites can be fierce. If you're marrying in this time frame, plan on looking for your ceremony and/or reception sites at least a year in advance.

Venue Options

Almost anything goes when planning your wedding. You imagination and budget are your limits. There are numerous unique venues available for holding your wedding ceremony, no matter where you live or choose to tie the knot.

SOME OF THE MORE POPULAR LOCATIONS

- **Stay put:** Holding your ceremony in the same location as your reception is a popular option. An adjacent room can be decorated to accommodate the ceremony, or a garden, patio, or terrace located on the same property can host the ceremony. There is often a fee associated with setting up a ceremony, even if you are having your reception at the location.
- **Fresh air:** Parks or gardens—public or private—are options that, provided you are marrying in the right season, provide built-in floral décor. When you hold your ceremony in a public location, be prepared for onlookers. If the idea of having strangers watch as you recite your vows gives you an uneasy feeling, look at more private options for this intimate moment.
- **Serene scene:** Water scenes are popular backdrops for a wedding ceremony. The beach or a lakefront can provide this scenery. A ceremony on a boat would also satisfy your quest for a waterfront wedding ceremony.

ESSENTIAL

When you select your location, make sure it complements your wedding vision. Fighting against the established environment will give you nothing but trouble. Ultimately, the wedding could end up looking like a stylistic disaster or cost you plenty of money to transform into your desired look.

The Ceremony Venue

Squaring away the details of your ceremony goes hand in hand with finding a reception venue, and should be one of your first and highest priorities. Competition for top ceremony sites in peak wedding months can be pretty fierce, so you're more likely to get the day and time you want if you start looking early. If you don't plan on having a long engagement, the best rule to follow is to arrange the date as soon as you possibly can.

Types of Ceremonies

One of your first decisions should be deciding what you would like the tone and style of your ceremony to be. To do this, you must take your own personal views on religion and marriage into consideration. Your upbringing and your family's views may also influence this decision. It is a good idea to acquaint or reacquaint yourself with some of the more common guidelines for wedding ceremonies. If you are not particularly religious or do not attend church regularly, you may want to examine some of the different types of ceremonies that are available to you. For more specifics regarding different types of religious ceremonies, refer to Chapter 10.

Below are some points to consider when making decisions about your ceremony, as they may impact your venue selection.

- **Civil ceremonies are nonreligious, and presided over by a civil or government official such as a judge, justice of the peace, a hired officiant, or a legally able friend.** Civil ceremonies can be as formal and dramatic as traditional church weddings, just without the limitations of religious laws or regulations. You will need a marriage license, and you may need witnesses; each state has different requirements, and you should always research what they are. If you opt for a civil or nondenominational ceremony, your particular house of worship may not recognize your union within its organization, although it is legally valid.

- **A nondenominational ceremony emphasizes religion without being associated with any particular religion.** It is often free of the structure and restrictions of traditional religious ceremonies, but does have a religious tone. The format of the ceremony typically resembles a traditional Protestant ceremony; however, customs and traditions from all religions may be blended into the ceremony. The reception venue—a boat; public spaces like a park, garden, or beach; and some nondenominational churches—are all possible locations for a nondenominational service. Nondenominational ceremonies are a popular choice for couples who do not have a strong religious background, have different religious backgrounds, are marrying in a place other than a house of worship, or want free rein to create their own ceremony.

- **An interfaith marriage is between two people from different religions.** Some religions will permit and recognize these unions; some prohibit them, and will not recognize the union. Interfaith ceremonies are usually held in religiously neutral locations. Many times, depending on the particular officiants involved, the ceremony may even be co-performed by leaders from both the bride's and groom's religion. Not all officiants will agree to these terms, so if this is what you want, be sure to ask.
- **Religious ceremonies will be held at a house of worship.** Many religious officiates who are affiliated with a house of worship (rather than for-hire religious officiates) will only perform ceremonies within the building walls. Religious ceremonies are more serious in tone and include secular reading and music. This type of ceremony is generally traditional and follows a tried-and-true format.
- **Commitment celebrations are often reserved for those who do not want a legally recognized union, but more often by same-sex couples in states where their marriage is not legally recognized (be sure to check you state's laws—this is an ever-changing situation).** Some more progressive houses of worship will welcome these ceremonies, but often, commitment celebrations are held in alternative locales.

Ceremonial Concerns

There are always questions when you plan a wedding. Before you make any final decisions, it is imperative to ask the right ones! That means getting into the nitty-gritty of setup, expenses, etc. When planning a vegan wedding there are a few extra technicalities to take into consideration. Don't get blind-sided; ask the right questions now to avoid trouble later.

Some of the following questions may pertain specifically to houses of worship and should be discussed with the officiant.

○ What kind of services does the facility provide (music, reception area)?

○ What fees are required for marrying in the facility?

○ What specifically do the fees include? Is there a security deposit?

○ What is the cancellation or postponement policy?

- ❍ Will the facility provide any decorations? Carpeting? Aisle runner? Ribbon?
- ❍ Are there restrictions on décor?
- ❍ Are there any restrictions on the kind of music you can have at the ceremony?
- ❍ Is a microphone or sound system available for the officiant?
- ❍ What are the rules regarding photography and video recording?
- ❍ Will you be dealing with a coordinator for the ceremony site over the course of planning the ceremony, or speaking directly with the officiant?
- ❍ Is there a bridal changing room?
- ❍ Are there any other weddings that day?
- ❍ Is there room to have a receiving line at the back of the facility? What about outside, in a courtyard or garden?
- ❍ What is the parking situation?
- ❍ Is the site wheelchair accessible?
- ❍ Is the site air conditioned?
- ❍ Is the site available for the rehearsal? At what time?

Exceptional Receptions

If you have never attended a vegan wedding, you may think you cannot have it all when it comes to your own wedding, but just because you are planning a vegan wedding does not mean you must sacrifice style or elegance for your ideals. Just be sure to choose a location that both of you agree on, whether it is a place with personal meaning or a place that you both feel comfortable in. Find a place that speaks to you. You want a location worthy of the occasion—this is where you exchange your vows and express your love for one another, so the setting should reflect the event.

Where to Go

You have numerous options when it comes to where you want to celebrate your reception. Each venue comes with its own special planning details and scenarios. Acquaint yourself with the possibilities and you can make an informed decision.

Home-Sweet-Home Reception

For many couples, the perfect solution to a reception dilemma is having a party at someone's home. If you're lucky, you, your parents, or someone you know will have a house and yard big enough to accommodate your reception. What better way to celebrate the most important day in your life than in the house where you grew up or the backyard where you used to play? Placed in a unique context and surrounded by family and friends, you'll have an incredible reception experience. You must be aware that if the guest count starts to climb, a home wedding can prove to be a logistical and budgetary challenge.

ALERT

Don't assume that having a home reception means your parents have to sweat in the kitchen all day preparing and serving food. If you're expecting more than fifty guests, it's best to bring in a professional caterer for the job.

Stay Right Where You Are!

Some receptions are held on the same grounds as the ceremony—the ultimate in convenience for you and your guests. Many churches and synagogues have a function room on the premises that you can rent without much fuss, at a cost much less than a commercial site. The reception is typically small and informal, and the menu is usually quite scaled back (maybe as light as cookies and punch or a small buffet).

FACT

Bear in mind that a site with a religious affiliation may not allow alcohol and may also restrict the kinds of music you can play at the reception. You have to seriously consider what style of reception you want if you choose to hold your reception at the church hall.

All in One

Having your wedding ceremony and reception in the same place is a very green option; it combines everything in one nice, neat package. No traveling back and forth between venues and no need for special transportation to get you from one place to another. Open your mind to what is in your area. You don't have to get married in a traditional wedding location—historical landmarks, museums, parks, gardens, art galleries, aquariums, old saloons, greenhouses—there are many exciting possibilities out there. Check with your local area chamber of commerce, your city's official website, your county parks, the web, and local bridal magazines to see what amazing possibilities lie in your own backyard. Look at local locations in a new light, and you may find the perfect place.

QUESTION

Are there advantages to staying close to home when planning a wedding?
A wedding in your own backyard is easier to plan and logistically organize. Managing vendors and detail is all much easier. It also saves the time and expense of traveling and cuts down on transportation-related pollution.

The Great Outdoors

An outdoor wedding in the middle of nature's glory seems to signify a love of the earth and a clean, fresh start to one's life. Beautiful flowers, sunny skies, big trees full of green leaves, or a lake with a waterfall in the background—how enchanting.

Locales and Challenges

You have so many choices—parks, botanical and organic gardens, nature preserves, and other welcoming sites. Just make sure to choose an area that won't be harmed by humans tromping and stomping all over the place. A pristine wilderness will be damaged by a wedding party trampling through the area, whereas a park, nature preserve, or garden is made for both natural preservation and human enjoyment.

Natural Challenges

However, any of these outdoor locations may pose their own challenges. Weather unpredictability being the biggest issue, you'll want to find a location that has options if the weather is bad—a pavilion, large building, or location where a large event tent can be set up to shelter everyone in case of rain.

Another big problem in the great outdoors can be pests, specifically mosquitoes. A truly green location will not use pesticides to control the bugs, so you may have a problem. Be sure to ask about natural pest-control solutions, and see what can be done to lessen the possibility of getting eaten alive on your wedding day. Citronella candles, lamps, and torches may be one possibility. Others may include using all-natural sprays and foggers before the event to shoo away the mosquito population, at least for the evening. The venue may take care of it for you, or it may be an expense you'll have to cover.

No matter where you get married, you'll want to know all the location's rules and regulations. The following are just some of the questions you'll specifically need to address for outdoor locales:

- Is there electricity available?
- Does the area have its own caterer? Can you bring in your own caterer? Can you have food at the location? Some natural settings may not allow food because of the resident animals.
- Are chairs, tables, and tents available? Is there an extra charge to use them?
- Does the location offer to set up and clean up, or do you have to do everything?
- Are candles allowed?
- What kind of noise and distractions may occur?

A big problem concerning outdoor weddings is electricity; you may not have access to any. If your event will be continuing into the late evening, you'll want some kind of light source. Renting a generator for power is one option. If you only need soft light, candles, oil lamps, and solar lights are some of your options. Strands of battery-powered LED lights or battery-powered flameless candles might also be possibilities. A big bonfire may be another fun option, depending on your location and what is allowed.

Getting Down to Business

Finding the right location for your wedding is the cornerstone of planning your event. After the research and legwork it requires to find that perfect place, you want to make sure there are no surprises. Make sure you have satisfactory answers to the following questions. Often the information can be found in the brochure or literature about the property, but the location manager should be able to provide answers to the following questions, and any others you may come up with.

Asking the Right Vegan Question

There are two sets of questions that must be addressed: the basics of locations and the vegan specifics. First, it is time to dive into the vegan-venue concerns and questions:

- Can you prepare an extensive vegan menu? Do you have any experience in serving a vegan event? Can we bring in our own vegan caterer? (See Chapter 11 for more on menu planning.)
- If we choose to go vegetarian, do you have any vegetarian specialties?
- If we choose to add an animal protein, can you provide grass-fed beef, free-range organic chicken, etc.? Is there an additional cost for this specialty?
- If we choose to serve an animal protein, may we designate certain tables as vegan friendly to keep meat eaters and vegans separate? If we chose a buffet, may we have two separate buffets; one for animal proteins and one for vegans only?
- If we prepare a list of vegan-friendly condiments will you serve those at the wedding? Do we need to purchase them or will you? Will there be an additional cost?

- Can you bake a vegan cake or other vegan desserts? If so, what types have you created before? If not, may we bring in our own vegan baker or dessert options?
- Can we remove any nonvegan-friendly items for the ceremony and reception area? (This may or may not be a concern, but clearly, if a venue has leather seating in their entry, you will probably want it removed for the event.)
- Who owns and operates the venue? (Do you want to rent a house for your event, only to find out that the owner is the hot dog king of the western United States?)

ALERT

Think about the décor in the venues you are considering. If a venue has an abundance of leather couches and dining chairs, antlers on the wall, photos of a cattle ranch, or a history that does not fit with the vegan life, cross it off your list right away.

Just the Facts

Regardless of any vegan aspects of the wedding, these are the basic catering questions you must get answers to before signing on the dotted line:

- ○ Is the site conveniently located?
- ○ What size party can the site accommodate?
- ○ What rooms are available?
- ○ How long is the site available for? Is there a time minimum that must be met? Are there overtime charges if the reception runs late?
- ○ Is there a dance floor? What size?
- ○ Does the site have a catering service? Can you bring in your own caterer if you wish?
- ○ Does the site provide tables, chairs, dinnerware, and linens? What about decorations?
- ○ Can the facility accommodate live music? Does it have the proper layout, wiring, and equipment?

❍ Does the site coordinator have any recommendations for setup and decorations? Can he or she recommend any florists, bands, disc jockeys, and such?

❍ Are there any restrictions regarding decorations, music, or photography?

❍ Are there any photos of previous receptions that you can see to get the overall feel of the place?

❍ What services come with the site? Waiters, waitresses, bartenders, parking valets?

❍ What is the standard server-to-guest ratio?

❍ What kind of reservation deposit is required?

❍ Will there be any other weddings at the site on the same day as yours?

❍ Is there a package plan? Is so, what does it include?

❍ Are gratuities included in the price you quoted?

❍ Is there any rental fee for table linens, plants?

❍ Does the price vary with the time of day?

❍ If it is an outdoor site, what alternate plans are there in case of inclement weather?

❍ Will the deposit be returned if you have to cancel?

❍ Does the site have a liquor license? Liability insurance? Are you required to show proof of liability insurance?

❍ What is the policy on open bars? If you do have an open bar, are you responsible for providing the liquor?

❍ Is there a corkage fee? If you're supplying your own liquor, some sites will charge a corkage fee to cover the costs of the staff opening bottles and pouring drinks.

❍ What are the drink prices at a cash bar versus hosted bar?

❍ What types of beverages are available?

❍ Is there an added price for garnishes for the bar?

❍ What is the layout of the tables? How many people does each table seat?

❍ Is there enough parking? Is it free? If there is valet parking, what is the policy on rates and gratuities?

❍ Is there a coat-check room? Will there be coatroom and restroom attendants? A doorman? What are the charges?

○ Are there changing rooms for the bride and groom?

○ Who pays for any police or security that may be required?

○ Can you see references?

Finalizing the Plans

Once you have solid answers to these questions, have evaluated your needs and wants, and have the facts and figures, you need to determine which site meets your needs and your budget. A deposit (usually a significant nonrefundable amount) will reserve the site you want. But don't hand over any money until you get a written contract stipulating every term of your agreement (specific costs, details, inclusions, exclusions, special requests). Signing a contract will also protect you from becoming a victim of escalating fees, which come into play when a couple reserves a site well in advance of the wedding date. Perhaps you've reserved the site in August for a wedding the following August. If you don't sign a contract specifying this year's prices, the site may try to charge you the new—higher—rates.

Get Out of Town

Maybe these countless options are just not for you; you have other ideas. You want to be whisked away to some romantic locale. And, heck, maybe you don't even want guests! There's a plane, train, or automobile waiting to transport you to the perfect location for your vegan wedding.

Destination Weddings

Destination weddings started as a hot wedding trend, but they are now a staple in the wedding industry, making them a very viable option for the soon-to-be wed. The location doesn't have to be exotic or sun drenched to meet the requirements of a destination wedding. A tropical island, an eco-resort, a grand English castle, or even your hometown all fall into the category of a destination wedding. If you must travel, it is a destination wedding.

It is really hard to say that there is a distinct advantage to having a destination wedding. It is just different than a traditional wedding. Some definite pluses include: a more intimate wedding, as less guests can usually attend; and the freedom of being away from your regular life. You may even be

able to find a location that truly embraces the vegan lifestyle and cuisine—
a huge benefit! If you do plan a destination wedding, remember, you are the
hosts for the three to four days the guests are there. You should plan activities, be a part of all the festivities, and provide travel and accommodation
information.

Planning Your Destination Wedding

It takes a slightly different approach to plan a destination wedding, and
you may encounter some obstacles. You must keep in mind some guests
will just not be able to fit travel into their schedules or the expense into their
budget.

> **BASIC STEPS FOR PLANNING A DESTINATION WEDDING**
> - Hire a wedding planner or select an all-inclusive resort as your desti-
>   nation to guide you.
> - Be sure there is a vegan community of some sort and access to vegan
>   food and supplies to pull off your wedding.
> - Scout the site before booking.
> - Inform the invitees of the travel arrangements and expenses via a
>   Save-the-Date notice.
> - Research the legalities for travel and marriage license requirements.
> - Arrange accommodations at a local hotel for the guests.
> - Plan a weekend full of activities, including transportation, and pre-
>   pare an itinerary for the guests.
> - Make arrangements for vendors traveling to the wedding.

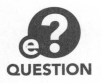
QUESTION

What are the challenges of planning a destination wedding?
Language barriers may make communicating with vendors, officials,
and locations difficult. Be sure to arrange for a translator. Be sure you
are working with someone who understands your vegan necessities.

You are not expected to cover the costs of the guests' airfare and hotel
accommodations; however, you may want to try and cover some costs for

the wedding party. You are responsible for the reception costs, the cost of any planned activities, and transportation to and from the wedding. Of course, if you have the means, covering the travel expenses is fine.

Who Needs Guests?

So, you're the kind of girl who hasn't been dreaming of her wedding since she was five. Maybe you are not interested in being the center of attention. Maybe you cannot imagine spending oodles of cash on one day. Maybe there are family dynamics that you just do not want to deal with on your wedding day. Well, eloping may be just what the doctor ordered.

An elopement is just the two of you heading off to get married, and surprising everyone when you return. You don't have to run far to elope, either. You can easily get married by a justice of the peace or at the courthouse where you obtain your marriage license. Some couples just hire an officiate to meet up with them at the local beach or park to perform a low-key ceremony. You will have to check into the local marriage license requirements to see if there is a waiting period or if you will need witnesses. When you make the big announcement, be prepared for shock, delight, and possibly some dismay from those, like your parents, who were wishing for the big wedding.

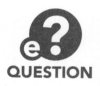

QUESTION

If we elope, can we have a reception to celebrate with friends?
A reception to celebrate with your friends is totally acceptable, and a great way to celebrate. Some couples have selected to surprise their guests by inviting them to a party and then making the big announcement. The more traditional route is to include the reception invitation with the wedding announcements so guests know why they are attending a party.

CHAPTER 6

The Write Stuff

Your invitation is the opening act of your wedding. It is a preview of what is to come, and can set the tone for your entire wedding. This paper wardrobe creates a unique look, but is it environmentally conscious? Are there better options? Are you thinking about skipping the paper altogether? Is that too modern? Or do you prefer to stick with tradition and select a beautiful assortment of stationery for your event? Luckily, you have options and opportunity to make your own statement.

Making the Change

Approximately 350 million wedding invitations end up in American landfills every year. Invitations have become increasingly intricate: outer envelopes, designer liners, overlays, ribbons, flowers, and embellishments galore! Etiquette and tradition dictate what you are supposed to send off in the mail. But, is it right for your circumstances? Fortunately, there are ways for you to create a vegan-friendly, greener invitation that (hopefully) won't end up in a landfill.

ALERT

Trees are the earth's principle means of processing carbon dioxide. The loss of trees and forests reduces our means of processing all the carbon dioxide that is released into the air. Global warming foes promote the planting of trees to offset the negative effects of carbon dioxide emissions.

Tradition Versus Change

It is a long-standing tradition that brides carefully select a complete invitation ensemble consisting of multiple parts. In fact many brides dream of the day their wedding invitations arrive and they can address and put them in the mail. Many couples are choosing to look at more environmentally conscious alternatives and reducing the number of parts in their invitations, such as forgoing the inner envelope or using a postcard for responses, but tradition dies hard. So, while not all couples are willing to go paperless, there are options you can consider to make your invitations vegan friendly and be kinder to trees.

Vegan Issues

Paper is one area where you are generally safe in your vegan ideals, but always check just to be sure you are using a vegan paper—with animal products in everything from gum to soap, you just never know. Sticking to eco-invites and other recycled and sustainable sources when it is time to select an invitation ensemble generally puts you in the clear. You will also want to look for vegan-friendly soy-based inks, and other inks that use no animal by-products. As a reminder, just because the invitations tout themselves as eco-friendly, be sure to inquire about the exact materials used so you can rest assured your selections are vegan friendly.

ESSENTIAL

If you want to tell your guests you are planning a vegan wedding, the Save the Date is the perfect opportunity. You can include an enclosure or a simple line at the bottom: "We are celebrating our love with a vegan wedding. For more details, visit our blog/website."

Eco-Invites

Choosing to show your colors—vegan with a dash of green—with your wedding invitations is a great option. There are many alternatives to traditional paper ensembles that make a unique and stylish statement while being kinder to the environment.

Recycled Paper

One option for change is to print your invitations on pretty recycled paper. Many printers now offer recycled paper and card stock. Some green printers only use eco-friendly papers and soy-based inks. Many times, you can find gorgeous handcrafted options from green printing companies with unique styles that your guests may not want to throw away.

FACT

According to Emily Anderson, author of *Eco-Chic Weddings*, more than 500,000 trees are destroyed each year for invitations, menus, table cards, and other paper items for weddings in the United States. To help lower this statistic, you can search for paper-free or recycled products.

You can also make your own invitations on recycled paper or card stock with earth-sensitive inks made from vegetable oil, linseed oil, hemp-seed oil, or soy bases. You can purchase kits you can use at home with your computer and printer. You could even try your hand at calligraphy and address your eco-invites with a gorgeous fountain pen.

By using recycled, handmade, and recyclable paper, you are saving trees from being cut down. Hopefully, by making your invitation unique and pretty, you may inspire your guests to hold on to your invitations instead of disposing of them in the trash. If you are still worried about the possibility your guests may throw your invitations away, you can include a note that says "Please recycle" with or on the invitation.

Tree-Free Paper Products

If recycled or handmade recycled paper isn't your thing, there are many more options. Tree-free paper is one eco-friendly alternative. The fibers from most plants can be made into quality paper products. Rapidly renewable resources such as flax and hemp can create quality paper. Experts believe the most effective and environmentally friendly resources for tree-free paper can come from otherwise discarded agricultural waste. Stalks and husks left after harvesting a main crop are perfect: corn, barley, oats, wheat, rice, rye, coffee-bean skins, sugar-cane husks, and even tobacco fiber can be made into paper. This method makes use of existing waste and turns it into something beneficial while saving natural virgin resources such as hardwood trees.

ALERT

When you mail out all those invitations, try to find old-fashioned moisten-and-stick stamps. New sticker-type stamps come on waxy paper that cannot be recycled. You can also ask for the invitations to be metered and stamped by a machine or by hand; just make sure the postage isn't being stamped onto peel-and-stick labels.

Some of the most popular alternative materials being used for paper-making today include the following:

- Bamboo is being used for everything from flooring to clothing and even paper. Bamboo paper and rice paper have been made on a small scale in Asia for centuries.
- Bagasse is the husk and pulp that remains after extracting juice from sugar cane; it can be processed into paper.
- Waste bark from banana trees can be made into paper. Banana-leaf paper is known as abaca.
- Coconut husks can be processed into thick, textured paper.
- Corn plant stalks, known as corn stover, can be made into excellent paper pulp comparable to North American hardwood pulp.
- Cotton paper can be made from old cotton rags and other recycled cotton material, cotton processing waste, or even fresh organic cotton fibers.
- Hemp paper is a superior-quality product. It is said that Thomas Jefferson drafted the Declaration of Independence on hemp paper.
- Straw fibers are very similar to wood and make great paper. At one time, the United States produced straw paper, but the industry no longer exists.

Hemp

Hemp is considered to be the best alternative to regular wood-pulp paper. It is said that the world's first paper was made from hemp, and until 1883, 75–90 percent of the world's paper was hemp. The Gutenberg Bible, Thomas Paine's pamphlets, and Mark Twain's novels were all printed on hemp paper. Hemp paper is stronger than wood-based paper and will last centuries longer. It does not crack, yellow, or deteriorate. Hemp paper does not require any bleaching and can be grown and processed with very little chemical use.

FACT

One acre of hemp can produce as much paper as four to ten acres of trees growing over a twenty-year cycle. While the trees have to grow for twenty to eighty years before they are mature enough to be harvested and turned into pulp, hemp can reach maturity in only four months.

Tree-free paper is not entirely a mainstream product yet, so it may be hard to come by at your local office supply store or printer. However, as with everything else, demand pushes supply up. As more people start asking for tree-free paper, mainstream stores will start supplying it to the general public. Until then, you can search in your local health food and natural-supply specialty stores and online.

Plantable Paper

If you want a very symbolic invitation that won't end up in a landfill, send invitations made from plantable seeded paper. The invitations will bloom just like your love for your fiancé. Plantable paper embedded with flower seeds is a great eco-choice. Depending on the seeds, the flowers may last for weeks or months after your wedding and no paper waste is left behind.

Many plantable papers are made from recycled or tree-free fibers and are embedded with seeds, so they are doubly and triply green. Not only were no trees harmed in the production of these papers, beautiful flowers will grow from them once they are planted. If you make your own recycled or tree-free handmade paper, you can add seeds to it at the end of the process while the slurry settles in the mold.

Consider using your postage on your wedding invitations or Save the Date to make a statement. Use the custom postage to create your own vegan wedding stamp or use nationally issued stamps that support animal rights and causes.

Ordering

Your invitations should be ordered anywhere from four to six months in advance (it all depends on the printing and details). This will allow enough time for the order to be processed and received, and the invitations assembled and addressed. If you are considering custom-designed invitations, you should allow yourself more time to account for the design process. Finally, always ask to see a proof of everything so you can proofread for typos and incorrect information before approving the final printing.

Here is a list of the basic information you should know as you begin researching wedding invitations:

1. Know the overall style and formality of your wedding—your invitations should reflect this.
2. Know how many invitations you need—you can usually count one invitation per household.
3. Have an idea about the wording—will your parent's names appear on the invitation? What about your fiancé's parents? Will you be using a poem or verse or other unique wording?
4. Confirm and reconfirm the details—be sure you have the correct ceremony start time, spellings of all names and locations, and addresses for ceremony and reception.
5. Know your response deadline—usually two to three weeks prior to the wedding. If you are using an RSVP service, you will need the company's designated phone number and website information.
6. Know if you are providing guests with a meal choice—you will need to have this indicated on the response card. You may or may not choose to include a simple statement such as, "We will be serving a vegan meal." This is totally optional, and not required. For example, you are not always told "We are serving chicken," when you are invited to a wedding.

Get 'Em in the Mail

Your invitations should be mailed approximately eight weeks before the wedding, with an RSVP date of about three weeks before the wedding. If you're planning a wedding near a holiday, mail out your invitations a few weeks earlier to give your guests some extra time to plan.

Details, Details

Once the guest list–making process is on a roll, make sure to keep yourself organized. Additionally, you must be thorough and complete when collecting the invitation information. There is really nothing worse than a guest receiving an invitation with their names misspelled, or having your beautiful invitations returned to you "Address Unknown."

You should check to make sure that all the following information is correct before mailing any invitations. If you're not 100 percent sure on any point, don't hesitate to ask someone who is in the know, or even ask the person in question.

- ○ Spelling of names
- ○ Titles (doctors, military personnel, etc.)
- ○ Addresses
- ○ Names of significant others

You Can Go Paperless

If you really want to reduce your footprint on nature and the Earth, and possibly prove your eco-centricity, go paperless. You don't need—although you may want—any of the fancy paper products wedding companies showcase. Not in today's electronic age.

You Did What?

Etiquette gurus may faint from the horror of it all, but you are a product of the green generation. The time-honored tradition of sending out printed invitations started before e-mail and the Internet even existed, and before we knew of the long-term damage we were causing the environment. Today's bride and groom have electronic advantages that past generations couldn't even dream of. Someone on the other side of the world is just a click away; as soon as you hit "Send," your invitation can be there, no postage or paper required.

You can cut down on paper invitations by e-mailing your Save-the-Date cards, or you can cut out paper entirely and send all the invitations themselves on the web. On some websites, you can create invitations and announcements quickly and easily with customized designs, your personal information, and even photos to include in your announcements or invitations. The sites also have many wonderful features that help you keep track of your address book, RSVPs, and much more.

Living in an E-World

The Knot, and several other wedding-planning sites, allow you to create a custom wedding website for free. Send everyone a link to your web page, and your guests can see all the information for themselves. Your page can include everything about your green wedding and all the information about when and where your wedding and reception will be.

Many companies offer premium website design and hosting services for a price, but The Knot, WeddingChannel, mywedding.com, and eWedding let you upload photos and lots of information completely free. Some sites allow you to keep the location and time password-protected so you don't get any unwanted crashers showing up at your intimate occasion.

ALERT

Even in today's electronic environment, Grandma and Grandpa and some of your other guests may not have computers and e-mail. Don't let this obstacle derail your paperless dreams. You can call everyone whom you can't reach electronically. This is a personal way to invite your guests.

There are a number of blog platforms that are also free, and you can easily update information and keep guests in the loop with a blog. And no need to worry about privacy—you can make your blog invitation-only, meaning only those you authorize to view the information can.

If you can't keep it completely paperless and must send out some paper invitations, be as simple and green as possible. You can always send a postcard on recycled or recyclable paper and request a phone or e-mail RSVP. Invitation companies now offer all-in-one unique wedding invitations with removable response cards so there are no envelopes and no excess paper waste. Send a few of those to the guests who require old-fashioned paper invitations.

Programs, Menus, and Place Cards

There is a whole selection of other printed goodies you may want for your wedding. Some brides find them to be essential elements of completing their wedding look; others consider them just more paper. That is a personal decision, as most of these printed items are optional.

Stationery Checklist

The list of what you can add to the stationery ensemble is long and varied. Depending on your type of celebration and the traditional or nontraditional route you are taking, here are some other items to consider:

- ○ Announcements
- ○ At-home cards
- ○ Boxes for the groom's cake
- ○ Ceremony cards (if your ceremony is in a public place)
- ○ Ceremony programs
- ○ Coasters
- ○ Cocktail napkins
- ○ Favor cards/tags
- ○ Matchbooks
- ○ Menu cards
- ○ Name cards (to let the world know if you are taking your husband's name, hyphenating, or retaining your maiden name)
- ○ Pew cards/within the ribbons card
- ○ Place cards
- ○ Rain cards (to notify guests of alternate plans in case of rain)
- ○ Table numbers/names
- ○ Thank-you cards
- ○ Welcome letters/itinerary for guests

Eco-Alternatives

That is quite a list; the question is, do you need it? Do you want it? Most of the paper products used in the name of weddings are just for décor or show. Some pieces, such as place cards, do have a purpose, and a ceremony program detailing the specifics of the event can be helpful, but generally they end up in landfills after the festivities are over. You can make a difference not just in the papers you select for these items but by having them serve double duty.

GREAT GREEN OPTIONS FOR PLACE CARDS AND FAVOR TAGS

- Use nonpaper products such as leaves, twigs, or small stones. Names or sentiments can be written on the surface for the reception, and they can be returned to nature afterward—no garbage created.
- Use recycled, handmade, or tree-free paper for them. Many of the companies that offer eco-fabulous invitations also offer eco-accessories such as guest books, favors, favor tags, place cards, menus, and even ribbons.

CHAPTER 7

Style for the Aisle

Your walk down the aisle is one of the grandest moments of your life, and without a doubt you should look and feel your best. The formality of the wedding will influence many of your decisions, but that does not mean you cannot inject some style and personality into your look or walk down the aisle in a fabulous vegan-friendly frock. But, remember, it is not all about you—your fiancé, the wedding party, and your parents are part of the wedding package, and are looking to make a stylish statement themselves.

Vegan-Friendly Fabrics

From the vegan perspective, it is crucial to find cruelty-free fabrics that have been turned into masterful works of art. Thanks to forward-thinking and socially responsible designers, it is possible to find an amazing selection of attire out there that is vegan friendly, organic, and/or crafted from eco-conscious fabrics.

Options

At first you may think, "How am I going to look like a million bucks in cotton?" You clearly have not explored the fashionable and exquisite options available to vegan brides and grooms in cruelty-free fabrics. From organic cottons to hemp silk to fabulous man-made fabrics, you will surely be able to find a dress or tux to put a smile on your face.

FACT

You may be able to get a gown designer to substitute silk fabrics for cruelty-free ones. There may be an additional charge, but guess what? Designers are itching to get into new, untapped, and up-and-coming markets all the time. Of course, some designers would not even consider altering their designs. Go ahead and ask; it's just a question!

Shopping is fun, but can be stressful if you don't know where to look, where to go, or what to do in order to get the vegan-friendly selection you desire. Begin your search online to find out what designers and manufacturers offer the selection you need. You can also get a great idea of styles as well as get acquainted with all there is available to you.

Fabric Selections

Rich and sumptuous natural cruelty-free fabrics can be turned into fabulous gowns. The bridal gowns that are available in natural, sustainable, and organic fabrics range from simple to stunning and can rival the beauty and elegance of any silk gown. There are a growing number of social- and eco-conscious bridal designers and retailers that offer ready-made bridal gowns or custom made-to-order gowns. Hemp, hemp blends, linens, and organic cottons will all serve your purpose and support your vegan beliefs. You may also want to keep in mind where fabrics originate and stick with fair-trade options.

Man-made and synthetic fabrics are definitely a viable vegan choice at a great price. Fabrics such as polyester, rayon, nylon, and vinyl (maybe not for a wedding dress!) are vegan fabrics. They may cost less than natural and organically grown sustainable fabrics, but they are often made from petroleum-based products that are terrible for the environment, and therefore for people and animals alike.

Natural Materials

Natural materials are good for you and for the earth. Choosing natural, organic, and sustainable fabrics for your wedding gown and other bridal attire is a great choice for the eco-conscious bride. Whether you buy the fabric and have a gown made for you or buy from an eco-friendly retailer, you won't be sacrificing style, beauty, or comfort.

Green designers and retailers offer gowns made from several types of natural fabrics. The most popular is hemp, followed by organic cotton-and-hemp combo blends. Bamboo, the newest sustainable fabric, is also making an impact in the wedding industry. Other sustainable fabrics include linen, canvas, twill, muslin, and jersey knits. Some may show up in wedding dresses, especially in a fabric blend, but many are not suitable for wedding finery.

Hemp

Hemp is a superior fiber known for being strong and durable. Hemp products will outlast competitive products made with other fabrics. Not only is hemp strong and durable, it is very comfortable. It wears in, not out. Hemp provides warmth and softness in a breathable material that is resistant to mold and ultraviolet light. It is nontoxic and great for those with sensitive skin.

FACT

U.S. laws prohibit the industrial farming of hemp because of its relationship to marijuana. Industrial hemp is only 0.3–1.5 percent tetrahydrocannabinol (THC), which is the substance that causes intoxication. However, it is legal to make hemp-based products.

What makes hemp perfect for wedding gowns is that it combines the soft elasticity of cotton with the smooth texture of silk. When hemp is blended with other fabrics, it incorporates the qualities of both.

Organic and Recycled Cotton

Cotton is the most comfortable and most popular fabric in the world. However, it is very hard on the environment. Organic cotton is growing in popularity because it is raised without toxins or synthetic fertilizers. Organic cotton is more expensive to produce, so it may be more expensive to purchase.

ALERT

Regularly grown cotton is the most pesticide-dependent crop in the world, accounting for 25 percent of all pesticide use. According to the USDA, more than 50 million pounds of pesticides are used on U.S. cotton fields in one year.

Organic-cotton clothing is available in many stores and online shops, and it is becoming popular to make green wedding dresses and other bridal attire from organically grown cotton.

Recycled cotton is another earth-friendly choice you can incorporate into your green wedding. Recycled cotton is made from fiber normally cast off during the spinning, weaving, and cutting processes. No harsh chemicals are used to process recycled cotton.

Lyocell

Lyocell, also known by the brand name Tencel, is a natural fiber made from wood pulp cellulose. It is the first new fiber in more than thirty years, and the first new natural fiber in much longer. While lyocell is a manufactured fiber, it is not synthetic. The cellulose is processed with a nontoxic, recyclable agent and is naturally biodegradable.

Lyocell is popular with formalwear because it drapes luxuriously and feels like silk. It absorbs dye well, and can be made into jewel-toned fabrics. Lyocell often appears as a hemp-lyocell blend in bridal wear. Like other natural fibers, it is comfortable, breathable, and resilient. Because of its sensuous texture and appearance, lyocell has become very popular with some of the top mainstream designer fashion labels.

When silk is made without killing the worms, it is called peace silk. Conventional methods kill the worms. Strict vegans will abstain from this fabric no matter what the outcome for the worms.

Bamboo

Bamboo is a sustainable product used for everything from flooring to sheets, and now it is making its appearance in the wedding dress. Bamboo fabric is spun and knit from the fibers of the bamboo plant. Bamboo can look and feel like silk, with a few key bonuses—it is machine washable and much more durable. Bamboo and bamboo-blend fabrics are appearing in bridal dresses at online retailers.

A sixty-foot tree cut for commercial use takes around sixty years to replace. A sixty-foot bamboo tree cut for consumer use takes less than sixty days to replace. Bamboo is a versatile plant that can be used for food, building materials, and decoration.

Man Made

Man-made fabrics such as polyester and rayon are vegan, and easily adaptable into formalwear and bridal wear. These are easily accessible options that have stood the test of time and are available at most retail locations.

The Bride's Ensemble

You may have dreamt about trying on wedding dresses since you were a little girl, but when the time comes and you are looking for "the one," you may feel a little overwhelmed and a lot pressured—it is a lot of work to live up to the dreams and visions you have in your mind. Make this experience a pleasurable one by working with a reputable bridal salon or seamstress. Professionals will be able to guide you through the process of finding your gown.

FACT

For the socially conscious bride, buying a dress from an organization that supports a charitable cause is the perfect choice. Making Memories (*www.makingmemories.org*) takes in used bridal gowns and resells them. The proceeds help make wishes come true for breast cancer patients.

Shopping for the Gown

You should begin shopping for your gown as soon as you solidify the style and formality of your wedding and set the date. Ideally, you'll order your gown six to nine months before the wedding, as some gowns can take that long to arrive back from the manufacturer or be sewn. You will also need to allot additional time for alterations. Some independent sellers or designers can turn around a gown in a few months, but to be sure you have the time to explore your options and get the gown you want, get shopping right away!

ALERT

Some shops can turn around a gown order in three months or less, but there may be rush charges that will hurt your budget. Shop early and shop smart to avoid this.

As you begin shopping, ask friends, family, coworkers, and your wedding planner for recommendations for a bridal salon. Also check the pages of the local phone directory, and if possible, visit a local wedding expo. Look to your favorite vegan boutique for a dress or for resources to the right vegan shop or designer. The shop owners may very well be able to direct you to a gown designer or company that can assist you in this special purchase.

Once you find a place you're seriously considering doing business with, ask for references from former customers, check with the Better Business Bureau (to verify that no complaints have been filed against the company), and look for reviews and comments online.

In order to receive the best possible service at a bridal salon, always call the salon and schedule an appointment. With an appointment you will have access to a knowledgeable bridal consultant who will assist you in finding the perfect gown, veil, and accessories. A few items you should take along when you shop for your gown are the proper undergarments, such as a strapless bra or bustier; shoes, in a heel height you typically wear; and any "must-wear" jewelry or accessories. In the end, you may be replacing some of these items with others, but it does give you a good idea of what works and what doesn't.

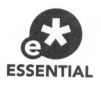
ESSENTIAL

When you call a salon to schedule an appointment, be sure to tell them you are vegan and make sure they understand the type of fabrics or designers you are interested in. You may even want to e-mail or drop off a list of acceptable fabrics prior to the appointment. You can even ask if they have a vegan salesperson to assist you.

The Gown

Buying a gown is about more than just what you want. You must take numerous factors into consideration when you make this major decision.

WHEN BUYING A GOWN, YOUR MAJOR CONSIDERATIONS WILL BE:
- **Fabric.** Of course, cruelty-free fabrics are your first priority, but there are other factors to consider. While many fabrics do double duty as warm- and cold-weather coverings these days, you should save heavy fabrics—like cotton or rayon velvet—for winter weddings, and choose from very light ones—like chiffon made from synthetic fibers—for spring and summer.

- **Sleeves.** Can you wear a sleeveless gown in the coldest months? Yes. Just bring along some kind of formal wrap in case you find yourself chilled. Likewise, if you want to wear long sleeves in July, make it happen.
- **Length.** If you're having an informal ceremony, a lacy suit is fine. If you're having an ultra-formal wedding, choose a floor-length dress with a very long train. For a semiformal wedding, either a tea-length or floor-length gown is a good choice.
- **Train.** There are many options for trains, from no train to formal cathedral-length options. Again, your choice all depends on the style and formality of the overall event.

Shopping Tips and Hints

When you head out to look for a gown, take only one or two trusted people with you, usually your maid of honor or bridesmaid and your mother. However, there are no rules about who should accompany you. Some brides have been known to shop with their grooms! You should also keep the following in mind:

- **Always talk to the manager of the shop.** Find out how long the place has been in business. You would hope that a disreputable establishment would not be around long.
- **Be careful of counterfeit gowns.** Some shops will tell you they carry brand-name merchandise, when in fact the gowns are cheap imitations, sold to you at a "real" price. Call the dress manufacturer or check online to verify that the shop is an authorized dealer for a particular designer.
- **Choose a delivery date for your gown that is several weeks before the wedding.** This should give you plenty of breathing room for alterations.
- **Make sure that the bridal shop doesn't try to get you to order a size that is much too big or small for you.** Don't expect the size of your wedding gown to be the same dress size you currently wear; bridal gowns are sized differently than ready-to-wear garments. Ask to see the manufacturer's size chart to see where your measurements fit in their sizing chart.

- **Don't allow the shop to use cloth measuring tapes.** Nonstretch fiberglass tapes should be used. Over time, the cloth begins to stretch, often yielding incorrect measurements.
- **Ask for verification of your order, and feel free to call periodically to check on progress.** Sometimes, the shops will hold your cash deposit for months before actually ordering your gown.
- **Get a written contract containing every aspect of your purchase agreement,** including delivery date, cost of dress, cost of alterations, and any stipulations for refunds if the dress is not ready on time.

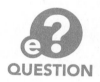

QUESTION

Should I bring a camera with me to the bridal salons?
Unfortunately, it's a prohibited practice in many stores. Bridal shops are brutally competitive with one another. They don't want you to have a picture that you could take to another salon—or to a dressmaker. Once you have put a deposit down, most will allow a photo.

If you decide to forgo the bridal shop route and have your dress made by a private seamstress, you should still guard yourself against the typical pitfalls. In addition, you may have to order your dress as much as a year in advance of your wedding, as that is how long it can take to make a gown from scratch.

Bridal Alternatives

If you're in the market for an alternative and possibly less expensive route for finding your gown, the bridal salon's discontinued rack is not necessarily your sole option. The following alternatives to high-end retail have all been known to pay off in major wedding-day savings. Just remember, always check for quality; there should be no stains, rips, or other major flaws.

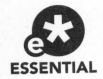

Heirloom and Antique Gowns

Antique and heirloom gowns can be significantly less expensive than new ones (but they can also be pricey, too!), and the added style and nostalgia they provide is beyond price. This is also a great use of resources and an eco-friendly option. Unless you're fairly petite, though, you may have a hard time finding one that will fit—women and sizing specifications were a lot different many years ago. Some brides may also wish to wear their mother's wedding gown. If this interests you, consult a skilled seamstress to see if this is a possibility.

Used or Consignment Gowns

Another way to get an inexpensive gown (provided you don't care if you're not the first and only person to wear it) is to shop the consignment stores and other bargain outlets for previously worn gowns. These dresses can be bought for a fraction of the original retail cost, and can be taken home with you that day. Of course, finding a quality wedding gown on consignment may require some tenacity and detective work on your part, since these don't come down the pike every day. If you're serious about taking the previously worn route, check out the classified section of the local paper, and don't forget about looking on the Internet.

Outlet and Warehouse Sales

Perhaps you've seen TV news coverage of a local warehouse's one-day wedding gown sale? Brides-to-be line up as early as six o'clock in the morning to get first crack at wedding gowns, many boasting top designer names, marked down as low as $100 each. It sounds great, but watch out—bargain hunting can be a full contact sport. In this maelstrom, women grab as many dresses as they can carry, irrespective of size, to increase the odds of finding a keeper. No one bothers much with dressing rooms, either, so if you're the modest type, be forewarned: Women try dresses on right next to the rack. If the stress and every-woman-for-herself atmosphere doesn't scare you off, you may very well walk away with a brand-new, top-quality gown. Make sure to double check the fabric used—you may get so excited you'll grab gowns made with fabrics like silk and with accessories like pearls and feathers!

ALERT

Every gown should have an FTC-required label showing the manufacturer/retailer, fabric content, and country of origin. A store may replace the original label with its own, but a label must be in the gown. It is illegal for a salon, bridal shop, or discounter to sell a gown without an FTC label.

Rent-a-Gown

Another increasingly popular way to find a gown is to rent one. Again, this option is not for someone who cares about being the first to wear the gown or who wants to keep it to treasure forever. Like a tuxedo rental, the gown is yours only for the wedding, then it's back on the rack for someone else. Through rental, a famous-maker extravaganza that would cost thousands to purchase can be rented for only a few hundred. The major kink in the rental game: If the gown you choose requires major alteration, they may not let you rent it. Think of how much valuable material would be lost in trying to fit a size 12 to a size 4 woman. After that, the dress could only be rented to very small women, a prospect the shop is unlikely to welcome.

FACT

If you have a good eye for fashion, an inexpensive alternative to a formal bridal gown is to find a suitable bridesmaid's dress. You may have to dress it up a bit with some lace, buttons, and so on. For a less formal occasion, this can be a thrifty and inventive way to go.

Accessories

You've found the perfect dress for yourself and the ladies, and you're thinking, "I'm done, I'm done, I'm done! Hooray!" Hold it right there, sister. You're not done. (Silly girl—you thought this would be as easy as finding a dress?) You need a veil and headpiece and all the little things to complete your ensemble. Summon up your strength, and pick yourself up off the couch. You're heading back into the trenches.

Although salons offer slips, nylons, bras, and shoes, the items they sell are often pricey. You're better off buying them elsewhere. The key is starting early enough so you can find what you need without being pressured for time.

What You Need

Completing the overall look for yourself or the ladies may require a collection of the following items:

- Slip
- Bra
- Hosiery
- Garter
- Gloves
- Shoes
- Jewelry (earring, necklace, bracelet)
- Veil
- Headpiece (tiara, headband, hairpin, florals, etc.)

Good-Looking Legs

Your footwear should be the same color as your dress (all whites are not the same). Choose a pair you can dance and stand in comfortably. Remember, you'll be on your feet for hours! Break them in by wearing them around the house before the wedding. One way to save a bundle on bridal shoes, if you're crafty, is to purchase a pair of plain, inexpensive shoes and decorate them yourself with lace, beads, or whatever suits you and your dress.

FACT

Bridal shoes are sometimes the worst offenders for vegan brides! Avoid leather soles and silk coverings and pearl details to ensure your feet are dressed as vegan as the rest of you. Vegan shoes of man-made materials are readily available at mass merchandisers and online retailers.

When it comes to hose, avoid opaque white stockings! Instead, go for the sheerest champagne, nude, or pale blush color you can find (depending on your dress color, sheer white or ivory are fine, too). Sheer stockings are classier looking and are flattering to legs, whereas opaque stockings can make perfectly fine legs look like tree stumps. Have an extra pair handy on the big day in case of disasters just before the ceremony.

Intimates

You'll want to purchase undergarments that work specifically with your gown. These may include a strapless or push-up bra, a corset, special tummy-reducing underwear, and a slip.

If your gown requires a petticoat, don't try to get away without wearing one for the sake of saving yourself a few bucks. The gown is designed to fall a certain way (that is, over a petticoat). If you go without the proper undergarments, you will have wasted the money you spent on the dress, because it just won't look right.

Dressed to the Nines

The men, and especially the groom (it is his day, too!) want to look their best on the wedding day as well. Typically, the groom and his attendants rent their formalwear and accessories. Vegans will have to be extra diligent, as many tuxedos are constructed with wool or a wool blend. Cotton and polyester options are available, but you may have to call around.

On the other hand, the men are not limited to rented formalwear, and in fact it may be easier and more cost effective to go another route. Depending on the locale and tone of your wedding, they can wear light-colored suits, thematic attire, or attire representative of your culture. It's up to you! The groom should go the extra mile by finding a smashing ensemble in a cruelty-free fabric.

FACT

Hemp not only feels wonderful and hangs well but is also a durable fabric that translates well to suits and tuxedos. Most hemp suits can be purchased for approximately the same price as renting a designer tuxedo, but you can keep the hemp suit to wear again.

The Groom and His Men

The men should determine their formalwear at least three months before the wedding. When renting from a formalwear store, a month is usually enough time to reserve the clothing in the off-season; it's better to be early and safe during peak wedding months (April–October). And to ensure you can find what you want and need for your vegan wedding, a little extra time never hurt. Obviously, the men should do business at a reputable shop that employs knowledgeable, helpful salespeople.

Formalwear Guidelines

Following is a guide to help the men dress the part:

INFORMAL WEDDING
- Business suit
- White dress shirt and tie
- Black shoes and dark socks (for winter, consider dark colors; in summer, navy, white, and lighter colors are appropriate)

SEMIFORMAL DAYTIME WEDDING
- Dark formal suit jacket (in summer, select a lighter shade)
- Dark trousers
- White dress shirt
- Cummerbund or vest

- Four-in-hand or bow tie
- Black shoes and dark socks

SEMIFORMAL EVENING WEDDING

- Formal suit or dinner jacket with matching trousers (preferably black)
- Cummerbund or vest
- Black bow tie
- White shirt
- Cufflinks and studs

FORMAL DAYTIME WEDDING

- Cutaway or stroller jacket in gray or black
- Waistcoat (usually gray)
- Striped trousers
- White high-collared (wing-collared) shirt
- Striped tie
- Studs and cufflinks

FORMAL EVENING WEDDING

- Black dinner jacket and trousers
- Black bow tie
- White tuxedo shirt
- Waistcoat
- Cummerbund or vest
- Cufflinks

VERY FORMAL DAYTIME WEDDING

- Cutaway coat (black or gray)
- Wing-collared shirt
- Ascot
- Striped trousers
- Cufflinks
- Gloves

VERY FORMAL EVENING WEDDING

- Black tailcoat
- Matching striped trousers trimmed with satin
- White bow tie
- White wing-collared shirt
- White waistcoat
- Patent faux-leather shoes
- Studs and cufflinks
- Gloves

ALERT

Be sure all the accessories are vegan, too. Silk finds its way into many ties, bow ties, and vests. Pearl and shell are frequently used for button covers and cufflinks.

The Little Guys

Most often, the ring bearer and trainbearer are little boys, but they probably enjoy being dressed like the big guys. In most weddings, the ring bearer and trainbearer are dressed in the same basic outfit as the rest of the men or in a slight variation of the outfit featuring knickers or shorts.

Of Course You Can Wear It Again!

Brides are famous for proclaiming, "You can wear it again." While the bridesmaids may not actually be able to wear it again, at least the days of ugly dresses are over. As any glance through a bridal magazine will show you, bridesmaids' dresses can be tasteful, elegant, vegan, and fashion forward.

The Bridesmaids' Dress

This is your wedding, and it should reflect your taste. Therefore, you do not have to consult with the ladies about the bridesmaids' dress you select (they knew this when they accepted your invitation). You can, of course, take their opinions into consideration, but they don't have final approval over what they wear.

Generally, the bridesmaids are dressed alike, but there is also the option of having the dresses differ in style. Going this route makes it a lot easier to make everyone happy, as a dress that looks great on one woman can look like a potato sack on another. You can also have only the maid/matron of honor wear a different gown, to make her stand out more from the other attendants. You should try to keep the color, fabric, and hem length the same (or nearly the same, depending on the case) to show some sign of uniformity.

Beyond being a vegan-friendly selection, keep the following suggestions in mind when shopping with your attendants:

- Check the formal dress section of a quality department store in your area before you go to a bridal salon. You may find appropriate dresses there that your attendants can wear again, and at a cheaper price than salon dresses.
- The attendants' dresses should complement your gown.
- Make sure the gown is one that flatters all the ladies in the wedding party. It may be your wedding, but they are paying for this dress; besides, if everyone looks and feels good in their dress, your photos will reflect that.
- Try to keep the cost of the gown within reason.
- If all of your attendants' shoes have to be dyed the same color, it is best to have them dyed together, to ensure an exact color match. Of course, it is more eco-conscious to find vegan shoes that do not need any dying.

The Flower Girl

Flower girls are a sweet addition to a wedding. The flower girl's dress can match the attendants' dresses or it can be completely different, but it should always be age appropriate. The flower girl may also wear white, either accented or not with a color to match the wedding colors. The dress may be short or floor length, according to the style you want. If you have trouble finding something, a fancy party dress is a good and inexpensive choice.

CHAPTER 8

Party Time!

As your glorious vision begins to come to life, you will also be the guest of honor at many a party. It is time for wedding season to officially begin. So, make that announcement, select that wedding date, choose your bridesmaids, and get ready to have fun and bask in the joys of being a blushing bride! As the wedding day draws nearer, it is time to start thinking about the other festivities that go hand in hand with a wedding celebration.

The Perfect Opportunity

The idea of others throwing a shindig may seem a little daunting. It is one thing for you to plan and orchestrate a vegan celebration, but what about leaving such a thing in the hands of others, especially nonvegans? Consider this the perfect opportunity to strut your vegan knowledge and introduce the party hosts and hostesses to a new way of thinking.

Planning Vegan Style

While the intentions of the host and hostess may be well meaning, don't expect that when they start planning they actually know how to pull off a vegan event. Without even realizing it, your dad may start planning his backyard BBQ for an engagement celebration, and really, it may be perfectly innocent. Ask him. His answer could be, "Oh, I did not realize all of the events should be vegan." When a person is not practicing a similar lifestyle, it may not even dawn on him or her.

Consequently, your foodie friend may be planning a wine and cheese party for the bachelorette party. Ask her and she may simply reply, "Well, vegans eat cheese!" This does not mean that any one of these dear people in your life are trying to undermine your event or values. Of course, those near and dear to you know you are a vegan, but in relation to planning a party and their lives, they may truly not know what that means.

Troubleshooting

Head off trouble before it starts, but do it in a sensitive way. After all, these are the people closest to you, and they want you to be happy and enjoy the wedding celebrations. If you are asking them to be sensitive, you need to be sensitive, too.

- Offer up a selection of vegan foods that you enjoy and suggestions and menus of vegan foods to the hostess.
- Compile a list of local vegan caterers and restaurants.
- Compile a list of vegan florists and décor sites.
- Purchase a vegan cookbook for the hostess if any of the parties are at someone's home.

- Find a vegan friend and offer up their assistance to the hostess in vegan planning matters.

The Engagement Party

Early in your engagement, the partying begins. Once all the major players have been notified, someone (usually your parents) will throw a party in honor of you and your fiancé. The bride's parents usually have first dibs on throwing the engagement party, but the groom's parents or your friends may want to throw a party, too. Have the parents confer about their party-planning ideas. This party can be as formal or informal as the hosts would like.

The engagement party is to give you and your fiancé an official coming-out party. It is also a chance for the families to bond with their newfound in-laws, and for your friends to get better acquainted with the other people in both of your lives. And, in your case, set the vegan tone for the wedding.

The Party Basics

The engagement party marks the beginning of wedding season! Although it is customary for the family of the bride to host some sort of an engagement party, it's perfectly acceptable for the family of the groom (or anyone else) to host such an affair—or do without one altogether, if you prefer. Many engagement parties nowadays are very informal, with invites made via phone or a handwritten note. The party is usually held either at the host's home or in a restaurant. Guests do not typically bring gifts to an engagement party.

The first toast at an engagement party is made by the father of the bride to the couple. This might be followed by a toast from the groom, who will tell everyone how happy and lucky he is to have snagged you. Anyone else wishing to offer a toast may then do so.

Showering the Bride

One great perk of following the traditional road to your wedding day is that you'll suddenly find yourself in the middle of a gift-giving storm. Although you won't be hosting a party for yourself, whoever hosts your shower (or engagement party, for that matter) will probably be looking for your opinion on any number of issues—the guest list, the menu, games. If the hostess is not a vegan or unfamiliar with the vegan lifestyle, you may be called on for more opinions and input than usual.

ESSENTIAL

Talk to a vegan friend and see if she is willing to work with the hostess of the party in order to prepare and present a vegan menu and celebration, so that you can sit back and enjoy!

Who's Hosting?

In the past, etiquette dictated that a bridal shower could only be hosted by your friends, not by family. This generally holds true for immediate family, especially the bride's mother. But it is not uncommon to find the groom's mother or family members, coworkers, or anyone else who is eager and so inclined wanting to throw a shower for you. The most common hosts are your bridal party, but who's to say which other generous (and ambitious) people might have a party up their sleeve(s)?

Typically, a shower is held either at a small function hall or in someone's home, depending on the size of the guest list. The guests are usually women, but your fiancé can come along for the ride if he wants. He probably won't be nearly as excited as you are about the pots and pans and measuring spoons and place mats, but you never know.

When?

Showers are usually held two to three months before the wedding date. If you absolutely cannot corral your most important guests within the confines of this time frame, shoot for a slightly earlier date (say, three-and-a-half months prior to the ceremony) or one that's a little closer to the wedding (but no more than a month before the big day). You're looking for a date within wedding range. A date that's too close, however, might set you up for feeling stressed over last-minute wedding details while trying to squeeze your shower in somewhere.

FACT

There was a time when the specifics of the shower—time, date, location, and so on—were kept secret from the bride until the last possible moment. These days, however, it's common—and in many cases, necessary—for the bride to take an active part in planning the festivities.

Who's Invited?

Making up a guest list? Check with your host(s) first and touch base on the budget. If the plan is for your shower to be a small, informal affair to be held in someone's tiny apartment, your list will obviously be much different than if your hosts are renting out a huge banquet hall. In either event, who should be invited, and who should be left off the list?

Any guest who is invited to the shower is automatically invited to the wedding. Period. You can't get around this one, and if you try to, you'll look greedy and insensitive. And even if you know you're sticking to this rule, it's in your best interest to make sure your hosts aren't inviting women who aren't on your wedding guest list.

Remember, all of this comes back to you. You can try to shift the blame onto the person who sent the errant invitation(s), but as the bride, you're the ultimate authority figure in this matter and the one who will be held responsible. If someone slips through the cracks, you're going to be forced to add another place setting at your reception—which isn't the worst thing in the world.

Shower Size

Often, different groups will host separate showers for the bride-to-be. Perhaps your bridesmaids will throw you a small shower; your coworkers will host another party; and the groom's family will have a third soirée for you. Is it all right for you to revel in such generosity? Of course it is.

Putting It Together

No matter how small the shower, the guests should be treated to a nice little party where they will dine, drink, and are entertained, with the event culminating in the grand finale—the gift opening. Throughout the shower, there will be chit chat and wedding talk, and yes, there may be shower games!

Food and Drinks

No matter the time of day or the number of guests, food and drink are required elements of the bridal shower. The shower menu can be as simple or as complicated as the hosts want it to be. If your shower is scheduled for noon, for instance, your guests will be expecting lunch. If, on the other hand, the party starts at three in the afternoon, lighter fare is more appropriate than a large meal.

Dessert to Die For!

You've fed them, but what's a meal (or a snack, for that matter) without dessert? Unless the guests will be having a sit-down meal, with a dessert served afterward, the sweets table should offer a wide variety of choices, which can be so-beautiful-you-hate-to-eat-them works of art or your basic cookies. Cakes, bar cookies, brownies, and fruits dipped in chocolate are easy desserts to prepare, and they're crowd pleasers, too.

FACT

Another featured dessert can be a shower cake. Your hosts can order a shower cake from a local vegan bakery, but they can also bake one themselves. It can be simple or elaborate, depending upon how ambitious and creative the hosts are feeling. Not feeling the cake idea? A selection of vegan cupcakes is fun and a perfect way to celebrate!

Let the Games Begin!

Everyone has a definite opinion on shower games: You either love 'em or you hate 'em. Unfortunately, your personal feelings and the opinions of your guests may be different, so in the interest of keeping everyone amused, showers often include games.

You might cringe at the idea of shower games, and if you're inviting a small group of women who feel the same way, you can encourage your hosts to do away with the games and the door prizes altogether. Just be aware that if your guest list includes ladies from an older generation, those games and prizes are part and parcel of a wedding shower, as far as they're concerned. Sitting around and drinking wine with you and your friends isn't going to fit their definition or expectations of what a bridal shower is all about.

Tracking the Gifts

During the gift-opening part of the shower, put someone you trust (an organized bridesmaid, your mother, a friend—but not your six-year-old niece) in charge of recording each gift and who gave it. Choose someone who can keep things organized even if things get hectic, so that when you sit down to write your thank-you notes, you won't come off sounding like a confused bride. Make sure the person charged with keeping track of who gave you which gift understands the importance of the task.

Bachelor and Bachelorette Parties

Traditionally, sometime before the wedding, friends of the bride and groom take them out (separately, of course) to celebrate the end of their single days. These parties are not mandatory, but your single friends might be disappointed if you don't want one. While the bachelor party has been around for a long time, the bachelorette party only became popular in the latter half of the twentieth century, probably due to the sexual revolution.

The maid of honor, together with the other bridesmaids, is in charge of the bachelorette party, while the best man and groomsmen organize the bachelor party. The organizer may ask all attendees for contributions to pay for the shindig, and since party guests are not expected to bring gifts, it's perfectly all right to do so, as long as all the invitees are told about the plans and financial arrangements in advance.

These parties were once held the night before the wedding, but now they're usually held a week or two before the ceremony, thus ensuring that the members of the wedding party will be fully recovered from their hangovers in time for the wedding.

CHAPTER 9

Giving and Receiving

You may be just starting a home and need everything from forks to hand towels, or you may be combining two households, and consequently have two of everything already. Don't worry! There are different registries for different couples. Perhaps you may want to use this time to open some eyes (gently), and encourage your guests to make a difference, through fair-trade, vegan-friendly products or by volunteering and charitable contributions. No matter the case, you have choices . . . and thank-you notes to write!

Gift Registry 411

A gift registry is a free service provided by many department, jewelry, gift, and specialty stores. The purpose of a gift registry is for you and your fiancé to compile a list of gifts you would prefer to receive at your wedding shower and the wedding itself. When friends and family go into these stores, pulling up your registry is as easy as finding the touchscreen computer that contains the information. Many registries are also available online, as part of a store's website. As each item is bought, it is removed from the list, helping prevent duplication.

FACT

A carefully assembled gift registry can help put you on the road to a beautiful, functional, and well-stocked home. It will also help direct guests toward organic cotton bedding and bamboo cutting boards rather than wool blankets and steak knives.

Which Stores?

You and your fiancé should put some careful thought into which store or stores you will register with. Make sure each store has a variety of quality items in the colors and styles you want. You might consider registering with a specialty shop, but remember that the point of the registry is to make gift buying as convenient for your guests as possible.

High on the list for a vegan couple is finding vegan-friendly companies and products to register for as well as companies and stores with ethical and fair-trade business practices. It all completes the circle of creating a cruelty-free, eco-conscious environment for your home.

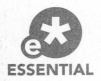

ESSENTIAL

It's best to register with at least one high-quality department store that is sure to have almost everything you need and have a national audience so that guests from all over can easily find a registry.

Even though you don't mind making the long haul to your favorite little store downtown, some of your guests might. What's more, smaller stores, though they may offer a bridal registry, may not be set up to offer the convenience of purchasing gifts online. While you may choose to register for a few household goodies in a small boutique, you may want to reserve the lion's share of your registry for a store that is easily accessible to the majority of your guests.

Before registering with a store, ask about the policy on returns and exchanges—you don't want to be stuck with duplicate or damaged gifts or nonvegan gifts. Make sure the store will take responsibility if you receive gifts intended for another couple and vice versa. Even brides with names much more exotic than Smith or Jones can share their names with someone else out there. If they've both got bridal registries at the same store, there can be a mixup.

FACT

To prevent receiving gifts intended for a bride with your same surname, make sure the store uses your groom's name and/or your wedding date as an additional point of reference when your friends and family log on to the store computer or the website to purchase their gifts for you.

Home Sweet Home

When the time comes to register for your wedding, you and your fiancé, armed with your vegan knowledge and tips, should decide what items you need or would like to register for. Many stores, as well as their online counterparts, offer complete lists and registry advice to aid in this process.

Plan and Prepare

Before you head to the store, you should discuss colors, styles, and preferences for housewares and décor for your registry. Once you have some of these details in place, you can decide which stores are right for you to register at, and then officially establish your registries. This will enter you into the store's system, and make your selections available for viewing by your guests.

Prepping for the Task

When making your wedding-gift list:

○ Shop with your groom so that you make choices together.
○ Consider registering at two stores (at least) to give a wider price range to your guests.
○ Discuss return policies with the bridal registrar.
○ Ask for a preprinted listing of gifts and household items the store offers.
○ List all pattern numbers and color choices.
○ Inform your family and friends where you're registered.
○ Have the store suggest that everyone send their gifts to your home rather than bring them to the reception.
○ Inquire with your insurance agent about coverage to protect the gifts while they're being displayed in your home.

On a final note, some salespeople/consultants mistakenly tell you to put the store's registry cards in all of your invitations. While it is acceptable to include this information with shower invitations, it is not okay to enclose these cards with engagement party or wedding invitations, as a gift is not a requirement for either of these events.

A Vegan Registry

As a vegan, you may wish to add a new dimension to the registry. Depending on where you live, you may not be able to do the across-the-board registering at any old store. You should be familiar with the products and stores that carry a selection of vegan-friendly merchandise. At larger (nonvegan) stores, you just need to take the extra step to ensure products and brands you choose are vegan friendly and/or not made with any animal products or tested on animals.

ALERT

If a guest purchases a gift that is not on the registry and not vegan friendly, do not make a big issue. Simply return the gift and send a thank-you note. This is not the time to get into a discussion of the pros and cons of veganism and "Why can't you just stick to the registry?"

Vegan Necessities

There are a few supplies you may want to register for that will definitely assist you in establishing your vegan home and cooking fabulous vegan meals:

- Juicer
- Food dehydrator
- Sprouting jars
- Specialty slicers
- Mortar and pestle
- High-powered blender
- Immersion blender
- Canning equipment
- Indoor grill
- Steamer
- Electric rice cooker

Lead by Example

Requesting that gifts be cruelty free and animal free is a given to you, but it may confuse some guests. There will be those that will question or possibly not even understand why they cannot give you a wool blanket, while others will be totally on board and understanding of your lifestyle. Be clear, and present the options to your guests so that they can make an informed and vegan-friendly decision.

To appeal to the gift giver in all the guests, you may want to think a little out of the box as well as incorporate some eco-friendly ideas into a gift registry. Some of these options include:

- Request that guests make donations to particular charities rather than bringing gifts.
- Register with the I Do Foundation or another similar site that gives a percentage of gift purchases to your chosen cause.
- Register with stores and select brands that offer vegan, local, fair-trade, handmade, organic goods.
- Do the work for the guests, and keep the items on your registry organic and sustainable.
- Go off the beaten path when you register. Consider gardening supplies for your own organic garden, park and museum passes that support culture and a cause, and memberships in local vegan or green groups, as well as subscriptions to socially conscious publications.

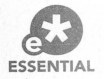

ESSENTIAL

Let your guests know about these alternative registry options via a wedding website, your wedding blog, in your bridal shower invitations, and through word of mouth.

Support a Worthy Cause

Being vegan can encompass so much more than living cruelty free, just as being green can encompass so much more than just saving the environment. Make your wedding day meaningful by supporting a worthy cause while you plan your big day and your life together afterward. This can be accomplished by supporting companies that are doing good things for their workers and their community, purchasing from businesses that donate part of their proceeds to charity, shopping directly from a charitable organization, registering for gifts from green stores, or requesting that donations be made in lieu of gifts.

A Typical Registry

Beyond the vegan necessities you select for your home, there are a host of other options. Take your time and browse through the store. Items you likely want to register for include a formal bone-free dinnerware pattern, a silverware pattern, glasses, pots and pans, linens, small appliances, and various other household items (measuring cups, candlestick holders, and so on).

When you decide on the styles, patterns, and colors you want, simply point the laser gun at the bar code and pull the trigger! If you're in the store without the bar-code guns, you may actually have to check the box next to the item and fill in the brand name and quantity in writing. (Such work to earn your gifts!) And even though you may feel awkward about it, don't be afraid to ask for a few big-ticket items like a television or DVD player. You may be helping friends or family looking to pool their money for such a gift.

ALERT

Be extra careful when selecting your formal and casual dinnerware. Many options are made with bone or contain calcium carbonate, a derivative of bone. There's no way you would serve your vegan meals on nonvegan plates!

A typical registry includes some or all of the following items (depending on what you need):

TABLEWARE
- Fine china (without animal by-products)
- Everyday dishes
- Silverware/flatware
- Glassware

LINENS
- Sheets and pillowcases
- Towels
- Tablecloths
- Placemats
- Napkins

COOKWARE
- Aluminum
- Enamel

- Glass
- Copper
- Microwavable cookware

More Possibilities

Couples and retailers are continually looking for and finding new avenues for bridal registries. Consider the following options if you really have all you need for your home:

- **Honeymoon registry.** A service offered, usually for a fee, by national travel companies, but may also be offered by your local travel agent. Guests help you "purchase" the honeymoon by contributing to this registry. The service should provide you with a list of all contributors and their gifts to facilitate sending thank-you notes.
- **Charitable registry.** Consider encouraging your guests to gift the charity of your choice in lieu of gifts for you. Through various charitable organizations, you can set up an online charitable registry that makes giving back easy.
- **Alternative gift registry.** A really unique website to register at is *www .alternativegiftregistry.org*. At the Alternative Gift Registry, you can let everyone know exactly what you want, even if it is something that cannot be bought in any store—such as Grandma's famous chocolate chip cookie recipe or a night on the town with your best friends.

This gift registry lets you request personal things that cannot possibly be assigned a price. You can also request regular items that you can link to outside the site, and you can list local craftspeople, artisans, and even local boutiques or farms that you would like your guests to purchase your gifts from. In addition to that, you can also request that your guests donate to certain charities instead of buying gifts for you.

Green and Eco-Friendly Registries

Even if you do not need or want a lot of new things, registering for at least several items that the two of you pick out together is a good idea. It is symbolic to choose things for your new life together. It is also a great bonding experience. Afterward, you can look at it and think "that's ours," not "mine" or "yours." It's good to have things that belong to the two of you together and are good for the planet!

Create a registry at a store that sells green merchandise. Choose eco-minded and socially responsible goods. There are many eco-fabulous retailers online that have wedding and gift registries. These web stores may carry a variety of items from towels to blankets to bowls to cutting boards. You can find stores that sell household products made from organic, recycled, and fair-trade items or furniture made from reclaimed and sustainable materials.

Register for sustainable household goods such as bamboo salad bowls and cutting boards; mini kitchen composters; garbage cans made from recycled tires; glassware and tableware made from recycled glass; art made from everyday recycled materials; organic bed linens made of cotton, hemp, or bamboo; luxurious organic terry cloth robes and towels; and so much more.

Giving, Receiving, Volunteering

While planning your big day, consider shopping for wedding supplies at eco-friendly retailers and charitable organizations. Many organizations offer favors and favor donations. There are also thrift stores that give their sale profits to good causes, such as Goodwill and the Salvation Army. When you are on the hunt for retro goodies and vintage inspiration, make sure to visit your local charity-run thrift shop to make the most of reusable style and green dollars.

If you are planning to make some renovations to your home or create some craftsy goodies for your wedding, check out your local Habitat ReStore. Operated by Habitat for Humanity, ReStores are retail outlets that sell used and surplus building materials, furniture, and interior design and décor accessories.

Charitable Donations

Instead of going all out and buying many things for your wedding that you really don't need, consider donating that money to charity instead. Instead of all those favors, place cards, confetti, and candles, donate a little something to the charity of your choice. The money will be well worth it. Charitable contributions can also be about donating yourself, your time, or your special talents or services. There are many ways you can contribute.

You can also donate your old stuff to charity. If it still has reusable life in it, chances are someone will take it. Getting ready to start a new life together is the perfect time to clean out some of the old cobwebs and get rid of clutter that has been piling up. There are charities that take anything and everything, and there are others that deal with only specific items.

Find something you are passionate about. There is so much to choose from—animal issues and animal rights, children's services, disease, the environment, homelessness, women's rights, poverty. You name it and there is an organization championing it that could use your help. There are several sites that can direct you to a worthwhile cause, including Charity Guide (*www.charityguide.org*), Network for Good (*www.networkforgood.org*), Charity.com (*www.charity.com*), and JustGive (*www.justgive.org*).

Charity Registries

Some organizations have created wedding registries for couples who would like to have their guests donate to a charity instead of or in addition to purchasing gifts. The I Do Foundation, in addition to their partner store registries, allows you to create a registry that consists of one or several of your favorite worthy causes that you would like your guests to contribute to.

FACT

JustGive.org also has a charitable wedding area that you can customize into your own unique charity contribution center. The World Wildlife Fund also has a wedding registry for nature-loving couples. At Heifer.org you can personalize your registry and decide which programs to help fund.

By encouraging your guests to donate to charity, you are showing the world that you care. Through one momentous occasion such as your wedding, you can inspire hundreds to donate money and perhaps even their time to a meaningful cause. They will tell others about it and inspire them to donate or create a charitable wedding registry of their own because they want to make a difference as well. One small action can cause hundreds and thousands of positive actions.

Get Involved—Volunteer

Make it all matter a little bit more by donating your precious and extremely valuable time. Volunteer alone, volunteer together, or get friends and family to tag along and volunteer as a group. Add to your ultragreen wedding by having charitable fundraisers or volunteer get-togethers as part of your prewedding parties. You could even include volunteering as a part of your bachelor or bachelorette party. Get your bridal party together and spend a day volunteering at a local Humane Society or animal shelter; hand out food at a food bank; give blankets, gloves, and hats to the homeless on a cold day; ladle out hot food at a soup kitchen; spend the day planting trees or flowers at a local park or school.

Finding Volunteer Opportunities

Organizations always need more volunteers than they can get. Schools, libraries, hospitals, senior citizen centers, children's organizations—so many need volunteers. ServiceLeader.org (*www.serviceleader.org*) has many great tips and ideas for volunteering. Network for Good (*www.networkforgood .org*) will help you search by state for volunteer opportunities.

HAVE A BRIDAL SHOWER OR PREWEDDING BASH THAT IS FOR A GOOD CAUSE:
- Have every woman invited to your bridal shower bring along an item of business clothing to donate to Dress for Success.
- Ask everyone to bring canned or boxed foods to donate to the local food bank.
- Get your entire wedding party together and spend the day working on a Habitat for Humanity house.

- Donate a Saturday morning to your local library and read to kids.
- Have an old-fashioned quilting bee. Project Linus (*www.projectlinus .org*) accepts new, handmade, washable blankets that can be given to children ages newborn to eighteen.
- Have a big barbecue/yard sale. Have everyone bring a dish to pass and something to sell in the sale. All money earned from the sale gets donated to the charity of choice.
- Have a wildlife party. Everyone who comes donates money at the door. All the money raised gets sent to your favorite wildlife organization.

If you feel as if you are being too pushy or feel that friends and family aren't into the volunteering thing, that's okay. You can volunteer on your own time without anyone else. There are many, many opportunities available.

CHAPTER 10

Getting to "I Do"

Are you finding yourself wondering, "Where and when does the 'I do' fit into this journey?" Well, rejoice, it is getting closer. Making the transition from engaged to married is a spectacular moment, and the wedding ceremony is an exciting and often nerve-racking experience that facilitates that transition. Depending upon your personal convictions, the style and tone of this transition can run the gamut from religious to strictly legal, but either way, there are many choices to make to enhance your ceremony.

Legalities

This is not the hearts-and-flowers-pretty-dress part of the wedding planning, but the fact of the matter is that marriage requires some legal forethought, and without it you can find yourself in a bind down the road, or end up with a marriage that may be less than legal. Don't overlook the legalities of getting hitched.

The License

What do driving, fishing, hunting, boating, selling alcohol, and getting married have in common? Legally, you need a license for every one of them. Admittedly, you're not threatening the public safety by getting married, but that license binds you as a couple in the eyes of the law.

FACT

If you are planning a same-sex marriage, you will have to continually check your local and state laws about the legalities involved. The laws for same-sex marriages are ever-changing with new legal issues and triumphs arising daily.

Give Me the License!

The criteria for obtaining a marriage license vary not only from state to state, but often from county to county within a single state. Before you head off to get your marriage license, find out how long the license is valid. There's no rule of thumb here. In some regions, the license is valid for several weeks, while in others it never expires.

General Concerns

Regardless of where you get married, you should be aware of some general guidelines for the marriage license. Every state addresses the following issues:

- **Paperwork.** You'll need some sort of valid identification (birth certificate, driver's license, proof of age, proof of citizenship). You must provide proof of divorce or annulment in the case of a second marriage.
- **Fee.** Every state charges a fee. Most are not outrageous ($30 is about average). Be aware that many states will accept only cash as payment.
- **Minimum age.** If you're fourteen and looking to get married in most states, you're out of luck, unless your parents agree to it. In most areas, you need to be at least eighteen.
- **Waiting period.** Again, this varies by state. Some states require a waiting period of several days between obtaining the license and saying "I do." In other areas, you can get the license and get married on the same day.

Your best bet is to make a call to your county clerk's office. There's a lot of information on the Internet, but not all of it is accurate or updated regularly. In this case, it's best to talk to a human being who has the most up-to-date information on the matter.

License Limitations

Just having a marriage license doesn't mean you are legally married. It means you have the state's permission to get married. To be valid and binding, the license has to be signed by a religious or civil official. When the ceremony rolls around, you'll give the license to your officiate. The officiant simply signs the license after the completion of the ceremony and sends it back to the proper state office. Now you're married. (Yay!)

Going to the Chapel

You must head to the chapel . . . or the hotel . . . or the park . . . or the courthouse . . . or somewhere to tie the knot. The type of ceremony will determine a lot of what goes into the final ceremony plans. There is no right or wrong answer (your mother may disagree, however), you just need to be comfortable, ask the right questions, and fulfill the requirements that are necessary.

Who's Going to Do It?

No matter the type of ceremony you choose, someone needs to marry you, to perform the act of uniting the couple. The officiant can be anyone from your family's pastor to an officiant-for-hire to a friend ordained (or deputized) to perform the ceremony to a spiritual leader. If yours is a legal union, as most are, you must be sure this person can legally perform marriage ceremonies in the country/state you are in. If you are a couple who cannot or choose not to have a legal commitment, this is not necessary; you can ask anyone you want to say a few words.

Meeting with the Officiant

Your first meeting with the officiant should clear up most of the technical details and give you the opportunity to ask questions. After everything is settled, the way will be clear for you to personalize your ceremony with music, scripture readings, special prayers, nonsecular music and readings, and even your own vows.

FACT

Your veganism will play little role in determining your officiant, unless of course you prefer to hire only vegan vendors to show support of like-minded individuals and organizations. Most officiants would be happy to incorporate your beliefs into the ceremony, even if they are not vegan.

Questions to Ask

What are the requirements (including any premarital counseling) for having you marry us/getting married in this church/synagogue? Even for-hire officiants may require premarital counseling.

- Is the date (and time) you're interested in available?
- Who will perform the ceremony? You may be close to a particular officiant, only to find that he or she is not available at the time you want.

- Are visiting clergy allowed to take part in the ceremony? If so, who will be responsible for what? Will you work with another officiant, such as a spiritual leader?
- Will you perform interfaith ceremonies? What are the requirements or restrictions involved?
- Will you perform same-sex ceremonies? What are the requirements or restrictions involved?
- Are there any restrictions on decorations? On music?
- Is another wedding scheduled for the same day as yours? Is there adequate time between the ceremonies so that you can have ample travel time?
- Are there any restrictions on where the photographer and videographer can stand (or move) during the ceremony?
- Will you be allowed to hold the receiving line at the site—at the back of the church or synagogue, for instance, or in a courtyard?
- You should also ask about the cost for the ceremony and for the use of church or synagogue personnel and facilities. This payment is typically referred to as a donation. It doesn't go to any single individual, but to the church or synagogue as a whole.

Learning Your Religion

If you're having a religious ceremony, consult with your officiant about premarital requirements as early as you can. Religions differ in their rules and restrictions, as do different branches within the same religion. If you're involved in your church (and/or have been to many weddings in it), you probably have some idea of what lies ahead. However, if you don't attend services regularly, or you're planning on marrying in your fiancé's church, you might not have the faintest idea of what's allowed and what's not.

During the meeting with your officiant, be sure to get all the details concerning rules and restrictions, your church's stance on interfaith marriages, any required commitments to raise children in your religion, and so on. Don't be afraid to ask questions. You want to make sure you and your place of worship are on the same wavelength on important issues.

Getting Personal

You've been to too many weddings that looked like carbon copies of each other. You desperately want to avoid falling into this trap, but how? Get creative. Use your imagination. Do some brainstorming with your fiancé or your friends. If you're attending some weddings in the near future, observe everything carefully. You don't have to copy another bride's ideas, but you can easily borrow inspiration and add your own spices.

Readings with Meaning

Nothing expresses the individuality and love of a couple like a ceremony filled with meaning. Readings are a popular way to personalize a ceremony, but you don't have to recycle the same ones you've heard at a dozen other weddings. If you're getting married in a church, your officiant will provide you with a list of recommended readings, most of which focus on some aspect of togetherness and marriage. You can choose the passages from the list that speak to you the strongest.

However, if you have a personal favorite passage that isn't included in the list of wedding readings, ask your officiant if it would be possible to include it in the ceremony. It may even be possible that he will be willing to include special song lyrics or a poem or build the sermon around your favorite biblical passage, as long as it incorporates an appropriate message for the occasion. If you are not marrying at a church or your officiant is more liberal, you may be able to incorporate nonsecular poems, love letters, and spiritual readings into your ceremony as well.

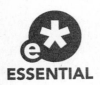
ESSENTIAL

If it feels right, ask the officiant to include a blessing of the animals or a passage about the earth or environment into the ceremony. This is a personal touch and pays homage to your veganism.

The Music

Music can add a new dimension to your ceremony, enhancing both its spirit and its meaning. You will have a broad range of choices here as well. Most officiants request that the songs you select be religious, but that doesn't mean you're restricted to music you only hear in a church. If you can find commercially released songs that meet the criteria, there should be no problem adding them.

If you have a friend or relative with a good singing voice or talent for playing an instrument, perhaps he or she can be persuaded to sing or play a special song. It would be best if they have experience performing in front of an audience; you don't want to have to give the soloist a pep talk just before the ceremony.

Symbolic Ceremonies

How else can you personalize your ceremony? Some couples like to acknowledge their parents by offering special readings or prayers that focus on family themes. Or, as you walk up the aisle, you could give a single flower from your bouquet to your mother and your groom's mother. Consider including a wine ceremony or a ceremony for the lighting of the unity candle. You might also take your vows by candlelight, and have the church bells ring as you are declared husband and wife.

ALERT

Be sure to consult with your officiant first about the possibilities open to you—once you know what's acceptable and what's not, it's up to you to be creative! Don't discount the officiant's input—he or she has seen a lot of weddings.

What Makes a Ceremony?

Each ceremony will differ slightly, but there is a basic guideline you can use for the items and the order of events traditionally included in a wedding ceremony. Depending on your officiant and type of ceremony, there are many ways to customize this outline by including readings, musical selections, and symbolic ceremonies.

SAMPLE OF A TRADITIONAL WEDDING CEREMONY

- The Prelude is the thirty minutes or so prior to the ceremony as guests arrive and are seated.
- The Processional signals the beginning of the ceremony. This is how everyone gets to their places. The mothers are seated, followed by the entrance of the officiant, groom, and groomsmen. The bridesmaids, followed by the ring bearer and flower girl, are next, and the bride and her escort are the grand finale.
- The Welcome is just that, the officiant welcoming the guests.
- The Giving Away or Recognition of the Parents is when the officiant will ask some version of "Who gives this woman to marry this man?"
- The Charge to the Couple is when the officiant confirms each party has come to marry of their own free will.
- During the Exchange of Vows, the couple recites their vows to one another.
- For the Ring Ceremony, the bride and groom will each give and receive a wedding ring symbolizing their union.
- When the Pronouncement is heard, you are officially married.
- The Recessional is the official exit from the church as a married couple. You and your husband will lead the recessional, followed by pairs of the bridal party in the reverse order in which they entered. The parents are also included.

ESSENTIAL

To emphasize the role of both parents leading their children through life, and to demonstrate the uniting of the families, both parents escort their children down the aisle in a Jewish processional. Take a cue from this ritual and invite both of your parents to walk you down the aisle, too.

A Few Words

You may want to formalize your commitment with something unique—something specific to your relationship or situation. If you want to write your own vows, check with your minister first to make sure that personalized vows are permitted during the ceremony. If, on the other hand, you're thinking, "I'm not writing any vows!" give it another thought. You get to stand at the altar once with your fiancé, and what better way to pledge your love than to do it in your own words?

Start at the Very Beginning

Where to start? Think about your relationship and the things that have the most meaning for each of you. For example:

- How do you, as a couple, define the following terms: love, trust, marriage, family, commitment, togetherness?
- How did the two of you first meet? What was the first thing you noticed about your partner?
- What was the single most important event in your relationship? Or, what was the event that you feel says the most about your development as a couple?
- Is there a song, poem, or book that is particularly meaningful in your relationship?
- If you share common religious beliefs, is there a particular passage of scripture that you as a couple find especially meaningful?
- Do you and your partner have a common vision of what your life as older people will be like? Will it include children and grandchildren? Take this opportunity to put into words the vision you and your partner share of what it will be like to grow old together.

Love Letters

Maybe this material isn't enough to get across the full meaning of what you want to say, or maybe you simply can't find the right words. Is it time to panic? Nope. Chances are someone else has said it already. William Shakespeare, Elizabeth Barrett Browning, your favorite musician—you may just need to find the perfect quote, poem, or song lyric to complete the mood.

Fortunately, there are many books in circulation of quotes compiled specifically for this occasion—look online or at your local library. Once you find a book of suitable verses, look in its index under "love," "marriage," "wedding," "husband," "wife," and other key words—these will direct you to appropriate passages.

FACT

Remember, the right way to compose your own wedding vow is your way. Look to your heart, recall a sweet memory, and connect with your spouse. Let your imagination be your guide to developing vows that are meaningful to both you and your partner.

The Second Time Around

Although certain celebrities may be experts at the remarriage game, there are some things you may have questions about if you're heading into your second (or third or fourth) marriage. There are a few rules of protocol to follow, but nothing you can't handle.

Clean Slate

If this is not the first marriage for either you or your fiancé, the main thing to avoid is the appearance of duplicating (or competing with) your previous wedding. You certainly don't want your fiancé to think you're trying to live in the past by recreating your first wedding. You want to start fresh.

If there was something you did at your first wedding that was particularly meaningful to you—if you wrote your own vows, for example, or if you carried roses because you and your mother grew them together in her garden—it's all right to include them in the second wedding. Things you should avoid recycling include the first dance music, readings, the dress (or any part of the bridal ensemble), the rings, and the reception site. Do things as differently as you can without crossing into foreign, this-is-not-the-wedding-I-want territory.

Shh! Keep It Quiet!

Many people believe that if they had a large wedding the first time around, they must keep things very quiet and subdued for a subsequent wedding. That's not the case, particularly if either of the marrying couple has never been married before.

In the past, second weddings were hush-hush, but these days they can include the same grandeur as a first wedding. The bride may still have a big wedding party and a big wedding dress; her father might walk her down the aisle; and there might be a slew of limos waiting for you and your attendants after the ceremony. You might also want to have the big reception with all the trimmings.

On the other hand, if you want to have a smaller second wedding, that's perfectly acceptable, and not the sort of thing that will raise any eyebrows. It's up to you and your groom to decide what's appropriate for the two of you.

Gifts or No Gifts?

Another point of concern for some couples is the issue of shower and wedding gifts. They feel that if family and friends gave gifts at the previous wedding, it's not fair to ask them to do so again. The answer to this dilemma is completely up to you and your fiancé. If the two of you are older and established in your lives, you might want to include a "No gifts, please" clause on your invitations. But if this is a first marriage for one of you, or if the two of you really would appreciate some help in starting your new life together, it's perfectly acceptable to have a shower and for guests to bring gifts to the wedding.

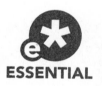

ESSENTIAL

As far as the ceremony itself goes, you should consult with your officiant about any restrictions or requirements surrounding the marriage of a divorced person. Once you've handled those issues, the ceremony can pretty much proceed as if it were a first marriage.

If you're a real stickler for etiquette, you can consult any number of books dedicated solely to the issue of remarriage. But these days, it really doesn't need to be that complicated. You and your fiancé should handle a remarriage in a way that makes both of you feel comfortable. If that means finding a middle ground somewhere between the big wedding he wants and the tiny wedding you want, then you'll have to play the game of compromise very carefully.

CHAPTER 11

Eat, Drink, and Be Married!

Eating, drinking, and being merry—or getting married—is what all this planning is all about. The food and drink is a major component of any wedding reception, and also one of the largest chunks of the wedding budget. But in your case, you are not talking about just any food; you need a vegan menu that will wow your guests as you celebrate this milestone in your lives. You have many options for creating an amazing and colorful menu that suits the festivities. So sit back, grab a glass of organic wine, and let's get eating!

Let's Eat . . . Vegan Style

Wedding guests are notorious for being food critics for a day. Perhaps it is because they have been waiting hours through a ceremony and other formalities; perhaps it is the anticipation of a wonderful meal; or sadly, perhaps it is because they have been to too many weddings with a subpar menu. When you take these preconceived notions into account, added to the fact that your menu will be vegan, you know the guests will be wondering, "What's to eat?" Well, consider this your opportunity to silence the doubters with a fabulous vegan meal.

ESSENTIAL

Whole-food chef and author of *Unprocessed*, Chef AJ assures couples, "People all across the world on a variety of budgets have wowed their guests with amazing creations from the plant based world. Once thought of as a hippie fad that was limited to the consumption of carrot sticks and sprouts, thanks to celebrities, vegan weddings are now in vogue and there have never been more talented chefs available to cater them."

The Star of the Show

Guests are notoriously critical of the food at any wedding reception. You also bear the burden of offering them a menu that they may not be used to—a new challenge, and a new treat if you do it right! Forget those ridiculous and unfounded grumbles about "too much tofu" or "rabbit food," and show them a thing or two about a vegan reception and a vegan meal.

ALERT

Serving any animal protein as part of the meal is not vegan at all, but it has been known to happen that a couple selects an organic, grass-fed beef (or the like) to appease some guests (and more likely, their family). This is a compromise not to be dealt with lightly. Do some soul searching before giving in—if it doesn't feel right, don't do it.

To really show off the beauty of vegan food, it is imperative to find a qualified professional caterer that is experienced in weddings, preferably an expert in vegan cuisine. If you can find a vegan caterer in your area, this is your best option, as they will know the ins and outs of vegan cuisine, and be able to prepare a menu including everything your heart (or mouth) desires.

When looking for a caterer, professional chef and vegan culinary expert, Chef AJ, suggests the following: "Find the closest veg-friendly restaurant or caterer near you. Then check it out. If you don't *love* the food when you sample it, don't expect it to magically be delicious on your special day. If there are no chefs that can do vegan food near you, don't give up! Many restaurants, chefs, and caterers can do amazing food if you ask them. Many will even let you provide the recipes. And if it's within your budget, with advance notice, many chefs will travel, so don't be afraid to ask."

However, if you cannot find a vegan caterer in your area, many professional caterers can and will accommodate a vegan menu. In fact, they most likely already have dishes on their menu that are vegan or can easily be converted to vegan. You may need to take a little extra care to ensure they really understand all of the essential ingredients to include and not include. A "regular" caterer can cater a vegan wedding and do a great job, so do not count them out; they may impress you.

ALERT

Visit Vegan Paradise (*www.veganparadise.com*) or Happy Cow (*www.happycow.net*) to find the vegan restaurants near you, and then go out there and start eating.

Guest Reaction

It is true that some nonvegan guests may be less than dignified in their responses when they hear you are having a vegan wedding. You should prepare yourself for a snide comment or two. It is not right, it is rude, but it may happen. As attendees at your vegan wedding, they should graciously accept the menu and move on, just as you have most likely accepted their carnivorous menu at their functions. Don't let your feelings get hurt by their insensitivity or lack of knowledge.

On the other hand, chances are good many of your guests, especially your friends, are willing and excited to try something new, and the fact that your feast is vegan won't faze them. Where you may encounter obstacles is with the older guests, or even younger ones who are just not open-minded (everyone has a few of those in their family, now don't they?).

Tempt Your Tummy

For most guests, the meal is where your vegan lifestyle will really be apparent. This is where they will sit at a table void of all animal products and the beloved animal protein they have come to expect. Rest assured, vegan cuisine can and will knock their socks off when done correctly. Vegan cuisine is gorgeous, as it comes in myriad colors and varieties, unlike the few choices you are given with fish, chicken, or beef. A feast for the eyes and senses!

Abundantly Satisfying

Vegan cuisine includes an amazing array of grains, pastas, tofu creations, vegetables, and fruits and when prepared correctly, guests will not even miss their beloved meat. Flavorful dishes are the key to outstanding vegan cuisine. Offer up a selection of infused oils, spices, and condiments to make the food come alive.

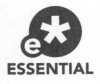

ESSENTIAL

"Whether you are doing passed hors d'oeuvres, a gala buffets or a sit-down dinner, vegan food can be as homey or as trendy as you desire. Vegan food also lends itself well to skewered food, whether it is fruits and veggies or seitan and tempeh. Remember, the sauce is boss, so make sure there's lots of exciting, bold flavors." —Chef AJ

Even if you are not a chef yourself, there is an abundance of resources available for you to find inspiration and recipes and help you plan your wedding meal. This is a great time for the guests to try new things, and the flavors will enhance the experience. This is by no means a comprehensive list of what you can offer, just a starting point to inspire you.

Hors d'oeuvres

Start the parade of tempting dishes off right with a selection of hors d'oeuvres that are fun, unique, and taste amazing!

- Risotto cakes
- Baked faux cheese in puff pastry
- Chilled veggie soups served in shot glasses
- Crudités with bean and vegetable dips
- Bruschetta
- Potato pancakes
- Tofu skewers
- Seitan fingers with dipping sauce
- Stuffed mushrooms
- Vegetable tempura

ESSENTIAL

You are already introducing your guests to a new culinary experience, so keep up that creativity from start to finish. Consider a raw station full of healthy, natural, raw foods and juices or even a pickled vegetable station consisting of cauliflower, beets, carrots, zucchini, and more for your cocktail hour.

The Main Course

After tempting the guests with a selection of hors d'oeuvres they will never forget, it is time to move on to the main course. Offer flavorful selections, tasty accoutrements, and a colorful menu to keep the guest happy and satisfied.

- Ravioli filled with squash or vegan soy cheeses
- Salads in all shapes and sizes (imagine the possibilities!)

- Fruit soups
- Veggie soups (think potato leek or carrot ginger!)
- Stuffed peppers and tomatoes
- Twice-baked potatoes
- Hearty rice dishes filled with nuts and dried fruits
- Quinoa accented with fresh herbs and infused oils
- Mushroom or vegetable roulade
- Herb-roasted root vegetables
- Beans (baked, mashed, salads, etc.)
- Couscous with chickpeas and sun-dried tomatoes

Sounds good, right? Again, this is just a small sampling of what can be offered. Who would miss the meat with a menu consisting of these hearty dishes? You may even want to go with a theme for your meal. Spanish, Cuban, Middle Eastern, and Asian cuisines have many, many options that translate nicely into vegan feasts.

Raw Options

If you want something truly unique and extraordinarily healthy, you may consider a completely raw-foods menu for your reception, or as part of the cocktail hour. Raw food isn't just salads and veggie trays. A raw food diet is filled with fruits, vegetables, nuts, seeds, sprouts, and fresh living juices that are packed with enzymes and nutrients to promote optimal health. It is all about the enzymes in fresh foods.

A raw diet made from organic produce is arguably the most environmentally sound and health conscious of all choices, but in today's fast-paced society, who has the time to sprout, dehydrate, ferment, and process their own organic, raw, living foods? However, if you have an expert raw chef or caterer in your area, this may be the perfect opportunity to try it out, either for prewedding parties or for your green reception.

Earthly Options

Most vegan caterers are already earth conscious; it is generally a part of being vegan. If you cannot find a vegan caterer in your area, look for an earth conscious one who uses organic products and respects the earth and environment. You may find only a few strictly organic caterers in your area, but many caterers offer organic menu options. The popularity of organic menus for weddings and other special events is growing rapidly, especially now that celebrities and celebrity chefs are joining the organic crusade.

How Does the Caterer Measure Up?

You can judge an eco-caterer on many levels, not just solely on the availability of an organic menu. Find out what her practices are. Does she recycle, support local farms and farmers, use local in-season products, buy organic produce, offer a wide variety of menus, or support fair-trade practices?

Organic is good, but supporting local farms and using fresh, locally grown, in-season produce can make a big difference as well. How green can it be if you want organic mangos in the middle of December in Maine? They might have been organically grown—thousands of miles away—but the carbon emissions produced to get them to your wedding feast make them not such an eco-friendly choice.

Toss It! Wash It!

Everything from the simplest details to the most complex choices can have an impact on the environment in some way. For example, what if you are having a big reception and you decide to use disposable place settings, napkins, and utensils? Would everything end up in a landfill afterward?

FACT

You can stop the excess landfill pileup by choosing to use reusable plates and tableware that you rent or purchase for the occasion. Alternately, you can buy compostable, biodegradable, disposable table settings made from sugar cane fibers, natural corn and potato starches, or bamboo.

You can be both eco-friendly and casual. If formal dinnerware won't fit in with your green wedding, retailers such as Kokopelli's Green Market (*www.kokogm.com*) and bambu (*www.bambuhome.com*) can help. Koko-pelli's Green Market sells compostable plates, bowls, cups, and cutlery; BambuHome offers beautiful single-use products made from bamboo that are supposed to biodegrade in four to six months.

Experts may argue which choice is better—reusable dinnerware requires water and energy to wash while biodegradable and compostable products have to be disposed of properly. It comes down to personal choice and what is the most convenient for you. Either option is greener than regular wax-coated paper, Styrofoam, or plastic disposable plates and utensils.

Service, Please

The menu you select for the wedding meal should reflect the time of day and formality of the event. For example, a four-course plated meal suits a formal evening affair while a cake and hors d'oeuvres reception better suits an afternoon event. When it is time to plan the menu, you must consider all of the elements of the wedding to make the right selections.

Options

When it comes to meal service, you have options; however, you must realize particular venues and caterers may specialize in one style or another, and not all caterers and locations will be able to accommodate all of the options.

- **The sit-down or plated meal is a traditional, and usually more formal, meal service.** It involves at least three courses: a salad/soup/appetizer, an entrée, and a dessert. Other combinations include a salad/soup/appetizer, an intermezzo, and an entrée. Of course, many upscale locations offer four- and five-course meals as well. It is important to make sure the venue/caterer has enough wait staff to serve all the guests in a timely fashion.
- **A buffet offers a display of food that guests can revisit as often as they like.** For buffets, make sure there are enough clean plates for multiple visits through the line, that the catering manager or emcee of the evening has a system for sending guests to the buffet to avoid long lines,

and finally, if it is a large wedding, that there are two or more buffet lines set up to avoid bottlenecking.

- **Food stations that serve made-to-order dishes are a popular option today.** You can generally expect to have at least three stations set up around the venue, each offering specialties (raw, pasta, salad, etc.). Due to the labor involved (chefs on hand at each of the stations), this is one of the more costly options.
- **Family-style meals are now being seen at both formal and casual weddings.** The caterer serves dishes to the tables, and the guests pass them around, serving themselves as if they were at your home.

ALERT

Should you choose to add a touch of dairy or other animal protein to an otherwise-vegan menu, be sure vegan and nonvegan options are clearly marked on stations and buffet tables. If you are passing hors d'oeuvres, those waiters need to know the difference as well.

Menu Checklist

When it is time to plan out the reception menu, review the Menu Checklist to make sure you are covering all of your bases and not leaving out any necessities or niceties.

MENU CHECKLIST AND CONSIDERATIONS
○ Bar (alcohol)
○ Children's selection
○ Coffee and/or tea
○ Dessert
○ Entrée
○ First course
○ Hors d'oeuvres
○ Kosher options
○ Nonalcoholic beverages
○ Raw options

Grilling the Caterer

You know you need food and beverages, but where to begin? What services do you need? All caterers are not created equal; most tend to have a specialty or style in which they shine. Vegan cuisine would be the specialty you are opting for, of course! You'll need to know some basic facts to get you started on your search for the wedding caterer, so here's the skinny on different types of catering services.

QUESTION

Do I need to hire a vegan caterer?
A good caterer, like a good wedding planner, can adapt and conform to serve any couple's needs. You do not need to hire a vegan caterer, but if it comes down to two caterers of equal professionalism and cost and one is a vegan caterer, that would be your best bet. Simply put, it is not essential but it is helpful.

Cater to Me

Catering can be basic or complex. It might involve two people in a kitchen making sandwiches and hors d'oeuvres for an at-home reception; a traveling company complete with cooks and a wait staff who will serve you at your rented reception site; or a full-service caterer supplying tables, chairs, linens, dinnerware, and a full bar and coordinating your whole reception for you, from flowers to photos.

Your head may begin to spin as you consider the options, but if you don't want your guests' heads spinning from hunger, settle down and take stock of the situation. Along with your budget, the type and location of your reception will help you determine the kind of caterer you need. After that, all that's left is to find out who can do it best at a price you can afford.

A caterer might be friendly, inexpensive, and cooperative, even downright artistic. But if his food doesn't taste good, RUN! Don't subject your guests to bad food for the sake of a great deal. Especially in your case, when guests may already be skeptical of what you are serving, be sure you hire a great caterer to fulfill your visions. Don't hire anyone without tasting the food first. It is standard to have a food tasting to finalize your menu.

Catering Options

The basic premise of catering a wedding—any wedding—is the same. You need good food to come out in a timely manner and a helpful wait staff. While your vegan ideals are essential in all components of the planning, when it comes to the food, it is probably the most essential element. The process for finding the right caterer is the same whether they are vegan or not. As you read through this section, realize how you deal with the caterer is universal. Depending on your venue and type of wedding, you will have many options for selecting a caterer. It is best to acquaint yourself with the simple facts about different types of caterers.

ESSENTIAL

If you hire a caterer that is not strictly vegan, you may want to prepare a list of vegan condiments and seasonings that are acceptable or that you prefer be offered. A good caterer will know that butter for the bread and cream for the coffee is not okay, but it does not hurt to cover your bases.

- **In-house (on-site) caterers** are provided by or contracted exclusively by your reception site, and are usually located on the premises. This is the type of service offered by all hotels and most country clubs. In-house caterers are already familiar with the particulars of the room, and can offer a lot of suggestions. On the flip side, because of the lack of competition, their pricing may not be as competitive, and typically you must select a menu from what is within their abilities (most are well trained and can meet requests).
- **Independent (off-site) caterers** come in all shapes and sizes. Your budget and needs will ultimately determine which style of food service and caterer is best for your event. Each offers a different degree of service, so there's no reason to settle for anything less than sheer perfection. The following are some of the main types you're likely to encounter:
  - **Food only.** These caterers specialize in keeping it simple—they provide food and food only. Everything else—everything!—has to be planned by you. This type of service can save you money in some

areas, such as allowing you to purchase the alcohol yourself to avoid the typical markups that accompany an open bar. While you may save money, you will invest time selecting and ordering rentals, hiring wait staff, and working through the details on your own.

- **Food and service.** This is the type of caterer that most people associate with a wedding reception. They provide the food, beverages, wait staff, and bartenders, and will usually assist with arranging for rentals as they pertain to the wedding reception (china, glassware, tables, chairs, etc.). Of course, somewhere in there you will be paying for these extra services.
- **All inclusive.** These caterers offer just about every item and service you could possibly imagine, as well as a few you probably couldn't. Many of these caterers have branched out into the event-planning business. Basically, if you choose to pay them for it, you can spend the months before your wedding in worry-free bliss, and leave the reception planning to the caterer. The price tag is typically higher for this type of caterer and you may be required to work exclusively with their preferred vendor selections.
- **DIY.** This is not a desirable option if you are planning a large formal wedding. However, in some situations, like smaller weddings or a potluck-style celebration, this option works just fine.

ALERT

If you're searching for a caterer for a wedding at home, make sure the catering service checks out the kitchen, appliances, storage, and electrical capabilities to ensure that everything is adequate. Your mother's tiny kitchen may be fine for the family, but how will it handle ten people trying to prepare and serve massive quantities of food?

Ask These Questions NOW

You have two sets of criteria a caterer must meet for your vegan wedding. The first speaks to your vegan fundamentals, and the second applies to any and all caterers. Your questions will evolve to more specifics once you book a venue, but in general, the following questions apply to most caterers. Once you've found a caterer with all the right answers, make sure to get every part of your agreement in writing.

VEGAN QUESTIONS

○ Do you specialize in vegan weddings? If you do not specialize in vegan weddings, why are you qualified/knowledgeable enough to cater our vegan wedding? Do you charge extra for vegan requests/changes?

○ How many vegan weddings have you catered? May we speak with one or two of those couples?

○ Are you experienced with vegan menus? What about raw selections?

○ Are you (speaking to the catering director or owner) a vegan or is there someone on your staff who is a vegan that may be able to over-see our specific menu?

○ What are my vegan menu options? Do you have predetermined menus, or may I create my own? May I offer up some special vegan recipes for you to recreate and include?

○ Do you offer organic menus, menus with organic choices, or cuisine made with organic ingredients? Will there be an extra charge?

○ Do you purchase locally grown foods from local farmers? Are the farms certified organic, or at least pesticide free?

Questions to Ask All Caterers

No matter what type of caterer you work with, there are a number of key questions you should ask before making a commitment. Vegan or not, these are basic and essential questions anyone who is catering an event on this scale should be able to answer.

QUESTIONS TO ASK ANY POTENTIAL CATERERS

○ What is your experience and catering background?

○ Do you have packages for the meals, or is everything priced separately?

○ What is the final food price? Caterers usually quote you an estimated price based on food prices at that time.

○ What types of meal services are offered? Sit down? Buffet? Stations? Family style?

○ When may we taste our selections? Is there a fee?

○ Do you provide bar service?

○ Is the catering service covered with proper insurance? (To protect yourself, you must make sure the caterer has the proper amount of liability insurance to cover property damage, bodily injury, and accidents that could occur during the wedding as a result of alcohol being served. Most venues require this and will not let the caterer work at the site without it.)

○ What will the ratio of staff to guests be? Will there be enough people to staff the tables? Will those people be dressed appropriately for the occasion?

○ Will you make provisions for guests with other special dietary needs? (It's only proper that you plan ahead for low-cholesterol or kosher diets.)

○ Will meals be provided for the disc jockey or band, photographer, and videographer? What do you serve them and at what cost?

○ What is the price difference between having hors d'oeuvres on display and having them served by the wait staff?

○ Can you provide a vegan wedding cake? How about a vegan dessert table?

○ Is there a cake-cutting fee?

○ Are beverages and desserts organic or local?

○ Do you provide reusable serving dishes, reusable real dinnerware, and cloth napkins and tablecloths? If you use disposable products, are they recyclable or biodegradable?

○ Do you provide any rental items, such as linens, place settings, barware, etc.? Are the rentals cruelty free (some china and dinnerware contain bone and bone by-products)?

○ Can you inspect rental items (linens, dinnerware, glassware)? Will you unpack and repack them for the rental company?

○ How do you charge for the wait staff's time? What about overtime?

○ Does the caterer's fee include gratuities for the staff? If not, what is customary?

○ What is the cancellation and refund policy?

○ What do you do with leftover food? Can it be donated to a local shelter?

○ Do you have references? (If you are not familiar with a caterer's work, ask for references.)

Stocking the Bar

Nowhere does it state that you must serve alcoholic beverages at a wedding. Just because someone expects something doesn't mean it is a necessity. You simply must provide the guests with refreshments, and nonalcoholic beverages are perfectly fine.

Guess what? Even your drinks can be organic and vegan! Beer, vodka, tequila, and wine are all being made in vegan varieties. Remember, not all beer and wine is vegan; there are animal products and by-products used in the filtering and manufacturing process of some varieties. To be sure you are serving a vegan beverage with your vegan meal, you must read the ingredients, and check out the Vegan Wine Guide, *www.vegans.frommers.org/wine*, for a list of vegan options.

Bar Lingo

When the time comes to select the type of beverage service you would like for the bar at your wedding reception, it is helpful to acquaint yourself with the options that are available to you. Be sure to consider your guest list, style of reception, and your budget to determine the style of beverage and/or bar service you will offer the guests.

FIRST DECISIONS

- Open bar versus cash bar. There is no argument here . . . a cash bar is a faux pas. Your guests are your guests, and should not be asked to pay for anything. Another popular option is to have an open bar only for the first hour of the reception. This will get things off on the right foot, and many brides feel this fulfills their responsibility.
- A full bar provides a complete selection of alcoholic and nonalcoholic beverages. For example, guests will be able to select mixed drinks, wine, or sodas at their pleasure.
- A soft or limited bar provides nonalcoholic beverages. However, many soft bars are now including beer and wine.
- A dry house is a beverage service that serves no alcohol of any kind for any reason.

Chances are good that the caterer will ask your preference on the quality of bar you would like to provide.

- A house bar consists of lower-priced brands the venue or caterer typically serves.
- A premium bar would be stocked with high-end brand-name selections.
- A deluxe or top-shelf bar serves top-of-the-line liquor of the best quality. You will have to do research for the brands you prefer (of course you may already have a preference), but many spirits are vegan with the exception of campari (contains cochineal) and some vodkas (which are passed through bone-charcoal).

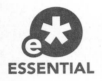

ESSENTIAL

Vegan does not stop with the meal. Double check with the bar that all garnishes are organic and vegan. It would be awful to see blue cheese–stuffed olives at your vegan bar! Then create a fabulous vegan signature cocktail to wow the guests!

Your Liability as a Host

Rejoicing with the bride and groom does not have to mean drunken reveling. But it does sometimes happen that a few guests go beyond the limits of common sense and wind up incredibly trashed. In recent court decisions, this has become a serious problem for both hosts and caterers. Be aware of your responsibilities.

Sorry, Junior

Liquor may not be served to anyone under the legal drinking age, even at a home party. Courts have ruled that hosts are financially liable when teenagers who are served liquor at parties in private homes become involved in auto accidents or criminal matters. Caterers and restaurants have been held to the same standard.

Sorry, Pal

If any of your adult guests are too drunk to drive but do so anyway and then have an accident after being served drinks at your party, the damage they cause is your responsibility and liability. As a good friend, you should call a taxi or find someone else to drive the car in these cases. Caterers and bartenders are also liable in this situation.

To avoid these situations, discuss with your caterer ways to limit alcohol consumption at your reception. Reliable caterers are happy to cooperate and to suggest options, especially since they are even more accountable than you are should there be an unfortunate accident.

CHAPTER 12

Let Them Eat Cake!

The wedding cake has evolved and transformed from its humble beginnings. It has also spun off many new ideas—cupcakes, dessert bars, mini cakes. The flavorful decadence of the wedding cake is celebrated by bride, groom, and their guests. Today's bakers are craftspeople, skilled at sculpting, creating, and baking up a wedding masterpiece. And yes, these masterpieces can be made gluten free, dairy free, and most importantly for you, they can bake up a vegan delight that everyone will enjoy.

And Then There Was a Wedding Cake

Wedding cakes are a long-standing tradition. They have evolved; now they are not just for cutting, they are a reflection of the couple's personality and the wedding's theme. They are magical creations of flour and sweet goodness. While cupcakes are still quite popular and dessert bars are closing in, there is nothing that will ever take the place of the wedding cake, its history, and this long-standing tradition.

History

Wedding cakes have been around since medieval times. In Rome, a loaf of wheat bread (*farreus panis*) was broken over the bride's head to symbolize hope for a fertile and fulfilling life. The guests ate the crumbs, which were believed to be good luck. Later, a variation of the custom found its way to England, where guests brought small cakes to the ceremony. The cakes were put into a pile, and the bride and groom stood over the pile and kissed.

Eventually, someone came up with the idea of stacking the cakes neatly and frosting them together, an early version of today's multitiered wedding cakes. Since then, the cake has lost most of its significance as a fertility symbol, and is seen primarily as a decoration and a tasty treat.

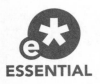

ESSENTIAL

Some couples follow the other cake tradition—the one where they smash each other in the face with cake. Whether this is a good idea is up to you. Generally, the cake is best saved for eating, not smooshing, and it is much more dignified to feed each other a bite nicely.

Preserving the Top Layer

Traditionally, the bride and groom preserve the top tier of their wedding cake to eat on their first anniversary. At first you may be thinking, "Yuck!" but if you preserve it correctly, the cake will be perfectly fine to eat as you reminisce about your wedding a year from now.

Check with your bakery, because some bakeries will now provide you with a small cake on your first anniversary in lieu of freezing your top tier. However, if it is your intention or desire to save the original cake, refrigeration alone isn't going to cut it. Taking the following measures should ensure that you'll have an edible cake come your first anniversary.

- ○ Wrap it tightly in plastic
- ○ Place it in a sturdy box
- ○ Wrap it in plastic again
- ○ Store in the freezer
- ○ When the time to eat your cake is upon you, thaw it in the wrappings for approximately twelve hours, then simply unwrap and enjoy!

Sweet Stuff

Modern couples are taking cakes to the next level with unique designs and gourmet flavors. Lucky for you, there is a whole new crop of vegan bakers who can whip up a vegan cake to rival any other. When you select a cake, you need a style, icing type, cake flavor, and filling. Pick your favorites, and enjoy a sweet moment with your new husband.

What's in a Cake

Cake is a sugary, buttery, floury mixture of sweetness. The nonvegan culprits in a cake are butter, eggs, and milk. While white flour may not be the healthiest ingredient, it is vegan. As far as white sugar goes, this is a gray area, but it is normally considered to be vegan. When a vegan creation is all mixed up, you can expect to find soymilk and soy butter, an egg substitute, and other ingredients to sweeten such as applesauce, brown rice syrup, and maple syrup.

In specialty markets and larger cities, most of these ingredients are readily available and easy to access. If you are having a large wedding, and therefore a large cake, confer with your baker ahead of time on what specific flavor you want, so she can order the correct amount, especially if your baker is not vegan or you are in a smaller town.

You've Got Style!

Each baker will have his or her repertoire of cake flavors—chocolate to tiramisu—and fillings—fresh fruit to white chocolate ganache—for you to select from. What you should understand before you get to that point is a little bit more about cake and icing options.

CAKE STYLES

- **Pillar:** Each tier of the cake is separated by pillars (clear, white, or colored). The space between the pillars may remain empty, or in some cases, accented with flowers
- **Stacked:** This cake appears to be stacked one tier right on top of the other, with no space showing between the layers.
- **Cascade or Satellite:** Each layer of the cake is decorated separately and placed upon its own pedestal, which stands independently of the others. The pedestals are of varying heights, so that it appears the individual cakes are cascading.

Traditionally, a cake was topped off with miniature figurines of a bride and groom. The cake topper, while still popular, has fallen slightly out of favor. Couples have used sparkling enlarged monograms, crowns, and even clusters of flowers to top the cake. Couples that do choose to go with a cake topper often look for vintage ones or even custom creations depicting various scenes or caricatures of themselves.

Designed to Perfection

The basic look and taste of the cake is just the beginning; it must look amazing and/or unique, too! To finish off the look of the wedding cake, depending on your budget and the skill level of the professional you hire, will be a variety of shapes—you are not limited to circular cakes anymore! Hexagons, squares, cakes sculpted to look like dragons, and even flaming cakes are the norm now. If that is not enough for you, the cake can be finished off with fresh flowers, sugar flowers, and other adornments crafted from edible and nonedible materials.

Icing on the Cake

You can achieve pretty much the same look with vegan frosting as you can with the standard sugary concoctions. Vegan frostings are every bit as beautiful, but the consistencies are slightly different than the typical. When you get down to making the final decisions on design, talk to your baker about which frosting type will hold up better in the temperatures in your area.

ALERT

Depending on the ingredients used, vegan frosting can be slightly more temperamental than standard frosting. Keeping it out of the direct sun or hot rooms for as long as possible may be necessary to ensure it is still standing when it comes time to cut the cake! Ask your baker for her expert opinion.

There are various types of icing, including:

- **Fondant:** Gives a smooth, clean look, and is very popular with the very modern and intricate styles of cakes today. It is a smooth, sheet-like icing that is rolled out. Traditional fondants include glycerin, which is an animal product, but a good vegan bakery will have a recipe sans the glycerin.
- **Buttercream:** Of course it will be a vegan soy butter that makes up this creamy sweet icing that is a traditional favorite. It can be flavored and spread on smooth, but does not give the sharp or defined smooth look that fondant gives.
- **Ganache:** A glaze of chocolate and cream (soy, of course) that is almost poured over the cake. It gives a shiny look with a consistency similar to the icing on a doughnut.

Want to add some more zest to the mix? These icings can be accented with tantalizing flavors—almond, orange, coconut, and more—to make them even tastier, more enchanting, and yummy!

ALERT

If you have your heart set on red icing or red velvet cake, look to beets or beet powder for that color. Many red food colorings contain cochineal extract, carminic acid, or carmine . . . meaning they contain dried bugs.

Cakey Goodness

The flavors you have available to choose from are almost limitless. Vegan bakers can create anything a regular baker can. Of course, there are the standard yellow, white, or chocolate cakes. But don't stop there; bakers are creative, and you can be, too. Consider some of these other fabulous options:

- Pumpkin spice
- Pineapple upside down
- Lemon pistachio
- Espresso
- Tiramsu
- Banana chocolate
- Almond rum
- Carrot cake

Don't discount the flavors that can be created using puréed fruits and vegetables. This may be an option you only want to move forward with if you are working with a baker experienced in this area of baking.

Fill Me Up

The filling in your cake is an element that can make all the flavors come together. The filling can be a simple fruit purée, decadent chocolate fudge, or a liqueur-infused cream. Almost anything you can dream up can be whipped up by your fabulous baker.

FILLINGS INCLUDE (THIS ONLY SCRATCHES THE SURFACE!):

- Apricot
- Raspberry
- Lemon
- Chocolate fudge
- Espresso mousse
- Vanilla bean cream

Finding the Right Vegan Baker

The wedding cakes of today are no simple affair; they may require a small army of bakers (and large chunks of time and money) to put together. Couples have grown to take great pleasure in designing edible masterpieces to display at their wedding, and bakers have risen to the challenge . . . most of them, anyway. Be sure you are getting the right baker for your wedding with these steps.

The Interview

To get a baker's undivided attention, call the shop to make an appointment. You can't pop in during their busiest time and expect someone to drop everything to talk business with you. This gives you an opportunity to get a feel for her skills and pricing, and ask any questions you may have. Some bakers do prefer to give you a sampling when you first come by to entice you! Just be sure to confirm these samples will be vegan.

ESSENTIAL

If you choose to use a baker that is not exclusively vegan, make sure you get answers to these questions: Can you bake a vegan cake? What is your experience with vegan cakes? How many vegan cakes have you made?

Where to Find a Vegan Baker

Of course, before you pop on over to the bakery, you need to know that the baker can produce a quality vegan wedding cake that looks and tastes good. There is an enormous amount of information on the Internet about everything, including vegan wedding cakes. Be sure to check out the web for reviews and general information on the bakeries and pastry chefs.

FACT

In recent years, bakers have become masters at reinventing the wedding cake into customized creations that not only look pretty but can accommodate varied dietary issues. As the number of children and adults with dairy and nut allergies has risen, not to mention the number of diabetics, bakers have risen to the challenge, creating dairy-free, nut-free, sugar-free, and gluten-free options.

If you are having trouble finding a vegan pastry chef in your area, here's a tip: Head over to the local health food store and look at their pastries—the in-house baker may be able to create a cake for your wedding. Additionally, ask the coffee shop or restaurant you frequent who they use to create their pastries.

Talking Cake

Like all other aspects of your wedding, you have some homework to do before you hit the bakeries. To help you get moving on your cake shopping, here's what you're going to have to do:

- Begin searching for a bakery at least six months before the wedding, possibly earlier if you are looking for an intricate or specialty design.
- Bring in magazine pages, photos, or books to show the cake designer, or view the bakery's sample books to find the right cake for you.
- Ask for taste tests of any style cake you're seriously considering.
- Tell the baker how many guests you expect.
- Find out how much of a deposit is required.

- Find out if the deposit is refundable.
- Ask about any additional delivery or rental charges.
- Ask whether there will be a fee for having the baker set up the cake at the reception site.
- Arrange when final payment for the cake is due.
- Order the cake.
- Get a written contract stipulating type of cake, cost, date of delivery, and any other important specifications.
- Arrange for the baker to arrive at the reception site before the guests to set up the cake.
- Decide where and how the cake will be displayed.

Questions to Ask

With so many options, coming to a final decision can be pretty hard. Here's a list of questions to ask your baker that might narrow things down a bit.

- ○ Do you use organic ingredients exclusively? Will you if we request them?
- ○ Can you make a gluten-free cake? A nut-free cake? A diabetic option? May we taste these options?
- ○ What size cake should you have for the number of guests you're having?
- ○ Can you have different flavors for different layers of the cake?
- ○ What choices are available in cake flavors and frostings? What icing style do you prefer to work with?
- ○ Do you specialize in any flavor, style, or size?
- ○ Do you offer a cake tasting? Is there a charge?
- ○ Is there a rental fee for tiers or separators?

Just for Him

In the very old days, the groom's cake was referred to as the wedding cake, and what we now call the wedding cake was known as the bride's cake. The groom's cake was traditionally a dark fruitcake—a symbol of the sweet life that lay ahead for the newlyweds—and the slices were packaged in monogrammed boxes as a wedding favor for each guest. According to superstition, if a single woman sleeps with the cake box under her pillow that night, she'll dream of the man she is to marry.

FACT

Groom's cakes are more common in the southern regions of the United States than they are up north, but being a Yankee doesn't preclude you from offering your guests a crack at a second confection. Just be prepared to explain the purpose of the cake to your guests who have never heard of this tradition.

Of course, as with all wedding traditions, this one has evolved with time. Since very few people actually like fruitcake, you should choose a flavor that will please the masses. If your groom is not vegan, and has gone along willingly with planning a vegan wedding, this may be the appropriate time and place to give him a little something special—his own decadent, nonvegan cake!

Tailored to Him

The groom's cake is supposed to give the groom his moment in the spotlight, so it should reflect his interests. Get creative here. If he's a hockey player, order a cake in the shape of a hockey stick or a puck. The groom's cake is supposed to be a little more fun than the wedding cake, so almost nothing is off limits.

Unless your groom is not a vegan and you want to give him his own cake, this cake should, of course, follow the same vegan guidelines as the wedding cake! Finalize the groom's cake by . . .

- ❍ Selecting a design
- ❍ Picking a cake flavor
- ❍ Ordering the cake
- ❍ Arranging for payment and scheduling the delivery
- ❍ Getting a written contract, just as you would with a wedding cake

Present and serve the cake at the same time as the traditional wedding cake. Or if you think that is just too much dessert (as if!), arrange for the groom's cake to be dessert at the rehearsal dinner.

Let Them Eat Dessert!

Perhaps you're the type of person who doesn't care for cake. You don't like six-foot-tall sugary sculptures, and you don't care what anyone says, you're not spending good money on one. There are alternatives to the traditional wedding cake. You and your baker can put your heads together and come up with something spectacular.

FACT

"The dessert can be anything from individual fruit cobblers to individual apple pies to peanut butter stuffed chocolate cupcakes. Nowadays, if you can think it, vegan chefs can make it. And who doesn't love chocolate? A chocolate fountain made with dark chocolate and plenty of fruit to drench it in is not only a healthy dessert option but decadent as well." —Chef AJ

Hey, Cupcake

Cupcakes came on strong about ten years ago, and have not slowed down one bit! Brides think their miniature size is adorable—a perfect bite or three of sweet perfection. Guests are still enchanted, and love the idea that they are being treated to something different. Cupcakes come in the same flavors as cakes, and can be filled with decadent goodness as well, and are considered no less formal than a cake. Stack them up on gorgeous stands and pillars to create a stunning masterpiece that can rival a grand cake, or they can be simply set out on a table, waiting to be devoured. The choice is all yours!

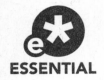

While many couples are ready to say sayonara to the cake, they start to feel nostalgic about the cake cutting. Who says you need to cut the cake for that traditional photo? You can do the same thing with a cupcake, cobbler, or sundae bar. If this really bothers you, order a small cake just for the two of you to cut.

Desserts to Die For

Forget the cake, forget the cupcake, let's skip to something new and different. Break out the cookbook, break out the creativity, and create a truly unique experience for your already unique wedding.

- **Fruit cobblers:** Imagine serving fresh-fruit cobblers of all sorts—apricot, berry, cherry. Top it with a crunchy, nutty topping and accent with a scoop of dairy-free homemade vanilla bean ice cream.
- **DIY vegan ice cream sundae bars:** Miniature cones and waffle bowls, vegan ice creams in all your favorite flavors, rich toppings including vegan brownies, peanut butter cups, and your favorite candies topped with a cherry make for a young-at-heart crowd pleaser with sophistication.
- **Doughnuts:** Who doesn't love a doughnut? Enough said. Stacks of warm, flakey doughnuts are sure to entice guests young and old.
- **Chocolate fountain:** This is a trend that has been around for a while, but for a vegan wedding it a fabulous option. Dark (healthy!) chocolate flowing, just waiting for the guests to dip fresh fruit and perhaps a few sinfully good treats into it!
- **Pastries:** Create a gorgeous display of coffeecake, danish, éclairs, turnovers, and cookies. Some couples do this in addition to a wedding cake, especially if their reception is scheduled to take many hours or run into the wee hours.

CHAPTER 13

Flowers, Décor, and More

You've seen the photos in fabulous magazines—lavish décor, grand themes, dramatic lighting. You want your wedding to be like that, too, and there is no reason you can't have it . . . or at least something close. The plans for those ultrafabulous weddings all started somewhere, and this is just the beginning for you. When it's time to dress up your wedding venue, garner inspiration from these fabulous creations. And even better, it can all be done while being socially responsible and vegan minded!

Flower Power

You could say that flowers are a wedding staple, and why not? They are beautiful to look at, lovely to smell, and add a touch of beauty to your décor. Flowers, no matter how grand or how simple, have a great impact on the visual presentation of your wedding. When used creatively, they are an effective means of enhancing the environment. While you do not necessarily have to worry about flowers being vegan, you should be concerned with the flowers being green. Now is the time to get some basic knowledge of what types of florals you should look for, find a professional florist, and go about ensuring your flowers have been grown organically.

ALERT

Be sure to give the florist a list of items not to use as adornments. It may seem simple enough, but many florists may not realize that silk ribbons and pearl buttons are a no-no for a vegan wedding.

The Floral Designer

When you first look for a professional floral designer, try to find one who is green or uses only organic florals and supplies. These stipulations should be high on your list of must haves. If you cannot find such a designer in your area, look for one that seems more progressive. How exactly can you do that? When you call them on the phone, ask the right questions, and get the answers you are happy with before meeting with them in person:

- Do you use organically grown flowers? All of the time? Some of the time? Never?
- If not, do you have access to organically grown flowers? And, can you/will you use them? Is there an additional fee?
- Do you have any suggestions for making my floral selection more eco-friendly?
- Do you have access to living centerpieces or décor so that nothing is being cut down?
- Will you refrain from using silk ribbon on the bouquets or pearl floral pins or anything else that is not cruelty free?

Gloriously Green

As you get acquainted with the basics in floral design, keep in mind you need to be concerned about where the flowers come from and how they were produced. And you thought they just needed to look pretty! Most brides dream of being surrounded by beautiful flowers on their wedding day, walking down the aisle amid an amazing floral fantasyscape. But how green is that? How much harm does that cause the environment and therefore the living creatures on the planet?

FACT

Cut flowers are one of the world's most pesticide-ridden crops. Since cut flowers are not considered an ingestible import, the USDA does not regulate the pesticide levels on them. Importers are free to load up on the chemicals to keep the flowers looking pretty and fresh. The flowers you choose can have a great impact on both social and environmental issues.

Solutions

There are green—or at least greener—solutions. Find florists that utilize green options such as buying fair-trade products, purchasing local flowers, using organic flowers, mulching and composting floral waste, recycling materials and packaging, and using natural, eco-positive products such as ribbons and paper made from tree-free, recyclable, and recycled materials. The choices you make can make a difference, both good and bad. The good news is that you do have choices. Look for florists that follow green practices and purchase eco-sensitive materials.

ESSENTIAL

If you can't find an eco-florist in your area, maybe you can encourage one to adopt more earth-conscious practices. If there are no local organic flower farms, point out to your florist that online organic retailers will ship large quantities of flowers for weddings.

The Organic Option

Organic farming works with nature by using natural techniques and old-fashioned methods to utilize the land and protect the air, water, and wildlife. Organic farming does not use harmful and toxic chemical pesticides or fertilizers. Organic floral farmers follow the same strict guidelines as organic food producers. It takes three years to transition from regular to organic farming, and the costs can be high. Plus, some don't believe that consumers really care whether or not products are grown organically, especially crops that are not food.

Due to the growing awareness of pesticide pollutions and dangers, many consumers do want choices. They want all of their products to be free of dangerous toxins, including their pretty flowers. As more people push for healthier solutions, more farmers will switch to organic growing. Let flower shops know you want organic flowers. In turn, they'll look for organic suppliers, and as regular suppliers start losing customers, they'll have to switch their practices to more environmentally acceptable solutions.

FACT

To know you are getting quality organic or sustainably grown flowers, look for USDA organic certification through Quality Assurance International. Also look for certification that the products are VeriFlora Certified Sustainably Grown.

Reduce, Reuse, Recycle . . . Reinvent!

When it is time to select your florals, remember some green, socially conscious and totally vegan-friendly essentials that help reduce and reuse elements and natural resources. Don't forget about recycling and reinventing other aspects of floral design to make your choices unique.

Three-R Thinking

To reduce the impact on the environment as well as save a little cash, choose floral elements that follow three-R thinking—reduce, reuse, recycle.

- If you dream of being surrounded by flowers on your wedding day, a ceremony held in the middle of a blooming garden might be among your top options for a location. It requires less decorating for you, and fewer flowers to buy.
- Renting large potted plants, flowers, and trees is another option. They can be used as decorations for both the ceremony and reception, and they'll go on to be used over and over again.
- Consider living floral arrangements. An assortment of plants and flowers can be planted together in containers. These can be used as wedding accents and reception centerpieces and décor. After the reception is over, guests can take them home and enjoy them indoors or plant them outside in a garden. The containers can also be donated to hospitals, nursing homes, and senior centers—any place that could use a little cheering up.
- Have the bridesmaids and flower girl carry nonflower elements such as decorative purses, vintage handbags, Southern-style parasols, Spanish- or Asian-style fans, or baskets full of organic fruit that can serve double duty at the reception as décor and food.
- Use nonfloral centerpieces such as soy candles, bowls of pretty rocks, or baskets full of fruits, nuts, or vegetables. If you are having a theme wedding, incorporate nonfloral theme elements into your décor that can be reused later.
- Keep it simple by only using flowers for what is really necessary: the bridal bouquet, boutonnieres, corsages, the altar arrangement (which can also serve as the bridal table centerpiece), bridesmaids' bouquets, and flower girl basket.
- Reuse the bridesmaids' bouquets at the reception. Invest in bouquet stands or clips that can be attached to tables.
- You can keep it extremely simple by using just one dramatic or exotic flower instead of a bunch of flowers as a bouquet. This could work for you and the bridesmaids, or you could carry the flower and they could carry something nonfloral. Calla lilies are perfect for this purpose.

Reinvent

To cut down on the amount of flowers you need to use in your bouquets, arrangements, and decorations, use your creativity and reinvent ordinary, everyday items, like natural elements as filler or focal points. Not only will lessening the number of actual flowers you use help save the environment, it can save your pocketbook as well. Fresh flowers can be quite expensive; minimizing the number you use can save you a small fortune.

Many natural elements may be found in your own backyard, or can be purchased very cheaply from local flower and herb farms. Many different things can be included in your bouquets and floral arrangements: leaves, twigs, berries, small filler flowers such as baby's breath, vines, ornamental grasses, herbs, and small fruits such as crab apples and grapes.

Small twigs can be tied in bunches and adorned with bright berries. Berries also make lovely accents in bridal bouquets nestled among the pretty flowers. In the fall, bundles of leaves can be grouped together for stunning bouquets and table centerpieces, and crab apples and grapes can be grouped together with fall leaves for beautiful centerpieces. You could even work them into a harvest bouquet symbolizing abundance and prosperity. Natural vines can be used instead of wires to wrap stems and twigs together.

Find the Right Florist

No matter what their specialty, professional floral designers should listen to your concerns and wishes. Don't hesitate to bring fabric swatches, pages torn from magazines, and books to convey the look you are trying to achieve to the florist. You should also be able to rely on them to offer advice on the types of florals that fit your budget and season as well as their perspective on trends and colors.

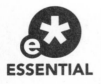
ESSENTIAL

You may have ideas, you may have visions, and yes the florist should listen, but she should also make knowledgeable suggestions as to when something is not right or going to cost you a lot more money than it should (for example, an out-of-season flower).

When you hire a florist, you should receive a detailed contract and proposal highlighting not only the amount of flowers you need but also the type of flowers, colors, and pricing as well as the setup and delivery schedules.

Local and Seasonal

The greenest and usually less expensive option you have for floral options is to use local and in-season flowers. Depending on where you live, different flowers may be in season at different times. If you live in a warm climate, some flowers may bloom all year long; in colder climates they may only bloom at a certain time of year. However, some organic flower farms have greenhouses and keep fresh flowers blooming all the time.

Here are the most popular fresh flowers you are likely to find during certain seasons:

- **Spring:** allium, anemone, apple blossoms, cherry blossoms, daffodil, freesia, iris, lily of the valley, lilac, narcissus, peony, ranunculus, sweet pea, tulip, violet
- **Summer:** allium, amaryllis, aster, calla lily, dahlia, geranium, gladiolus, honeysuckle, hydrangea, liatris, orange blossom, peony, rose, sunflower, zinnia
- **Autumn:** amaryllis, anemone, aster, calla lily, dahlia, some types of narcissus, marigold, sunflower, zinnia
- **Winter:** amaryllis, daffodil, hyacinth, mimosa, tulip, evergreens
- **Year round:** alstromeria, aster, baby's breath, bird of paradise, calla lily, carnation, daisy, eucalyptus, fern, freesia, gardenia, gerbera, gladiolus, iris, ivy, lily, orchid, rose, statice, stephanotis

Questions to Ask

After you have researched florists and found a couple you want to interview for your wedding, make an appointment to meet and discuss your overall needs. Use this list of questions to assist you in your selection process.

❍ Do you use organic flowers? If not, will you? At what cost?
❍ What is your specialty or style?
❍ Do you have arrangements that will fit my budget?

○ Do you have a portfolio of previous weddings and events we can review?

○ Can I have a list of references?

○ Can you match or complement the color scheme of my wedding (bring color swatches)?

○ Will you visit the ceremony and reception venue to get a feel for what type of flower décor is needed?

○ How many weddings do you handle on a given day/weekend?

○ If we reuse flowers from the church at the reception, can you assist with transporting these arrangements?

○ What is the cut-off date for making changes to our order?

○ Is there a delivery fee?

○ What is the cancellation policy?

Floral Checklist

Who needs flowers? Where and what type of flowers do we need? Simple questions to answer if you use the following checklist.

FLOWERS FOR THE WOMEN

THE BRIDE
○ Bridal bouquet
○ Toss bouquet (optional)
○ Floral headdress/flowers for hair
○ Going-away corsage
○ Other _____ _____

BRIDAL ATTENDANTS
○ Matron of honor
○ Maid of honor
○ Bridesmaids
○ Flower girl basket
○ Floral headdresses/flowers for hair (optional)
○ Other _____ _____

FLOWERS FOR THE MEN

○ Groom's boutonniere
○ Best man's boutonniere
○ Groomsmen's boutonniere
○ Ring bearer's boutonniere
○ Other _____ _____

FLOWERS FOR FAMILY AND HONORED GUESTS

○ Bride's mother
○ Bride's father
○ Groom's mother
○ Groom's father
○ Stepmother(s)
○ Stepfather(s)
○ Grandmothers
○ Grandfathers
○ Mothers' roses
○ Aunts, cousins, special friends, godparents
○ Other _____ _____

FLOWERS FOR WEDDING HELPERS AND PARTICIPANTS

○ Officiant
○ Soloist
○ Readers
○ Instrumentalist
○ Guest book attendant
○ Gift attendant
○ Hostess
○ Other _____ _____

CEREMONY SITE

○ Aisles
○ Aisle runner
○ Altar floral spray
○ Arch/Canopy
○ Candelabra

❍ Petals for aisle
❍ Pews
❍ Other _____   _____

RECEPTION SITE
❍ Bar
❍ Cake (if desired)
❍ Cake table
❍ Centerpieces for tables
❍ Cocktail tables
❍ Drapes, garland, or greenery
❍ Flower petals for tossing
❍ Gift table
❍ Head table
❍ Miscellaneous tables (place card, gift, and guestbook)
❍ Plants, trees, shrubs
❍ Restrooms
❍ Sweetheart table

REHEARSAL DINNER
❍ Centerpieces

Au Naturel Decorations

Stay on the vegan and eco-track by choosing fabulous decorations that range from natural elements such as twigs, rocks, flowers, and greenery to new and trendy green options such as artful centerpieces made from recycled glass, metal, or a variety of other items. Create big impact and big style with natural décor that pleases the eye and maybe even the palate!

Natural Decorations

You may want to let Mother Nature take center stage when you are decorating for your wedding. Many natural elements can be transformed into elegant and stylish decorations. Use the seasons to get the most out of what is naturally available.

Using green objects is truly eco-friendly because no extra resources are being used, especially when you use found and wild objects straight from your backyard—wild grape vines, blooming crab apple branches, nuts and acorns, fruit, and rocks. Open your eyes to the abundance that is all around you. If you'd like to venture further from your backyard, just choose wisely, and don't stomp all over someone's property or go hacking up their carefully tended landscaping.

ALERT

Balloon releases used to be popular at weddings, but balloons are potentially harmful to wildlife. Unsuspecting animals can often eat balloons or get tangled in the ribbons, sometimes with fatal consequences. You can still enjoy balloons at your wedding—just hold on to them and make sure they are properly disposed of.

The other great thing about using décor straight from nature is that everything can easily be returned to nature if it isn't taken home or eaten. Vines and branches can easily be mulched, and any perishable food items can be composted. Rocks can be returned to the stream or put in a garden.

Centerpieces

Centerpieces are among those seemingly must-have wedding-reception decorations. The most common types of centerpieces are those that incorporate flowers, candles, or a combination of both. You can quite easily use flowers and candles in many green centerpieces, or you could consider more unusual green options for your eco-extravaganza. Centerpiece choices can be as simple or as complicated and as varied as the couples choosing them.

Follow your three basic green guidelines (reduce, reuse, recycle) and you could come up with something no one else has done before. Some great green centerpiece ideas are:

- Pots of edible herbs or wheatgrass
- Pots of planted flowers guests can take home and plant

- Assorted topiaries, made from fresh or dried flowers, herbs, and other materials
- Natural wreaths laid flat on a table with a candle in the middle
- Bulbs planted in tall vases
- Small containers grouped to form a larger central display; this works great with small square containers or vases that can be pushed tightly against each other
- Apples, oranges, pears, peaches, or other fruits in tall, clear vases
- Trendy and chic vintage items
- Anything you choose made from recycled materials
- Vintage candy dishes and bowls filled with yummy treats
- Rented, borrowed, or secondhand bowls with floating candles in them; these look very elegant when placed over a mirror tile because the reflected light is soft and romantic
- Rented, borrowed, or secondhand vases filled with a single flower
- A potted minitree that can be taken home and planted
- Extremely eco-fabulous: favors that multitask as centerpieces

Borrowed Style

Many couples feel the look of their wedding stops with the wedding flowers, but other decorative elements such as lighting, rentals, and specialty linens can greatly impact your wedding look as well. Beyond basic party rentals (which you may or may not need depending on your venue), are a huge variety of fun extras that make your décor pop! You name it—sofas, coffee tables, tents, even movie props—you can have it . . . for a price.

Necessities

Most hotels, country clubs, and established wedding venues have all the basics you need—china, glassware, staging, etc. Most likely, you will only need to rent if you want something above and beyond what they are offering. If you do want to include something other than what your venue is offering (i.e., fancier, more elaborate, more unique), ask the site manager if they work with other rental companies that can supply these items. Often, through the venue, you will be able to upgrade certain items such as chairs and linens for just a few dollars more (each); much less than renting them on your own.

ALERT

Double check with your venue or caterer about what type of dishes they use or provide. Some dinnerware is made with bone or calcium carbonate, and it would be a shame to serve a vegan meal on plates made from animals. Look for earthware or stoneware.

Rentals Checklist

If you do need to organize rentals for your wedding, it can be a little confusing and possibly overwhelming. Most major rental companies have knowledgeable representatives that are there to help you. Look for a company that will offer this more personal service. If you are trying to outfit your entire event with rentals and don't have a wedding planner, you may be able to ask your caterer for assistance and advice.

RENTAL CHECKLIST

TABLES
- Bar
- Cake table
- Dessert or coffee
- DJ
- Food service (prep, buffet, etc.)
- Gifts
- Guest tables
- Guestbook
- Head table
- Place cards
- Sweetheart table

CHAIRS

❍ Ceremony
❍ Cocktail hour
❍ Highchair (for children)
❍ Reception

LINENS

❍ Chair covers
❍ Linens for each of the above tables you must rent
❍ Napkins
❍ Overlays
❍ Table skirting

FOOD SERVICE/PLACE SETTINGS

❍ Bread plate
❍ "Butter" dish
❍ Cake/dessert plates
❍ Cup and saucer
❍ Dinner plates
❍ Forks (salad, dinner, cake)
❍ Hors d'oeuvre plates
❍ Knife
❍ Salad plate
❍ Salt and pepper shaker
❍ Soup bowl
❍ Spoon (soup, dinner, coffee)
❍ Sugar and creamer set

GLASSWARE

❍ Additional barware
❍ Bar glassware
❍ Champagne flute
❍ Pitchers
❍ Specialty glasses (i.e., martini)
❍ Water glass
❍ Wine glass/glasses

MISCELLANEOUS

○ Aisle runner
○ Arches, gazebos, chuppahs, or columns (for ceremony)
○ Caterer supplies (consult with your caterer for a complete list of their specific needs and what is/is not included with their services/pricing)
○ Ceremony sound system (consult with entertainment)
○ Chafing dishes
○ Dance floor
○ Furniture (lounge chairs, sofas, coffee tables, etc.)
○ Ice buckets and tubs
○ Lighting (décor)
○ Lighting (utilitarian)
○ Podium or stand for officiant at ceremony
○ Portable restrooms
○ Potted plants/trees/shrubs
○ Serving pieces
○ Staging
○ Tenting
○ Trash cans

Questions to Ask

○ What are the delivery charges? How and when does overtime begin?
○ What are regular delivery hours?
○ Are you familiar with the site?
○ When are the rentals dropped off? Picked up?
○ How are the rentals priced?
○ When do you need a final count for the items?
○ Is a deposit required?
○ Is there an additional security deposit (i.e., for specialty or custom items)?
○ When is the final payment due?

Mood Lighting

Lighting has been a popular addition to high-end events for some time. It has now become increasingly popular for weddings of all budgets. The lighting need not be extravagant; even simple touches can make a huge impact on the look and feel of your wedding.

Candlelight Romance

Love is in the air, and nothing says elegance and romance like the soft, mesmerizing glow of candles. Choose candles made from natural soy or vegetable-based wax. Regular wax candles made from paraffin are not a very green option because they are a petroleum-based product, and beeswax is definitely not a vegan option!

Many natural and health food stores—not to mention boutiques, craft stores, and malls—carry candles made from soy and other vegan options. The concept has caught on quickly and now many online retailers offer wide varieties of soy candles.

ALERT

If you are not purchasing the candles yourself (or making them), be sure the florist or rental company will be providing soy or nonanimal-based candles.

Other soft lighting options include olive-oil and hemp-oil lamps. Not just any old oil lamp can be used with olive or hemp oil; they have to be designed a certain way and made for use with that specific oil. However, they can be rather hard to find. Check with green home goods stores for your options.

When choosing to use candles or oil lamps to light up your event, make sure that the location allows them; some places do not allow any open flames. Also be sure that fire extinguishers are easily accessible, especially if alcohol will be available. You never know when someone might get a little tipsy and clumsy.

If your location does not allow the use of open-flame candles or lamps, you can get the same effect from beautiful battery-powered flameless LED candles. Many can be found in grocery stores or online. You can find a wide variety of flameless LED candles—even some that are rechargeable—at smartcandle.com. Strands of LED lights also offer beautiful energy-efficient lighting. Get great deals on them right before or after Christmas when they go on sale.

Types of Lighting

Event lighting is very different than the standard lighting at a venue. Event lighting includes everything from washing the walls with color to spot-lighting guests' tables to your monogram floating around the dance floor. For these lighting services, you will need the services of a professional lighting designer. Also, be sure to talk to your venue/venues about restrictions and lighting capabilities before you go forward with these plans.

The term "gel" is still used by the lighting industry in reference to the acetate sheets used for lighting. At one time these gels were made from gelatin, but now they are made from man-made materials such as polyester or polycarbonate.

Some typical lighting choices include:

- **Uplighting:** Light that is projected onto a wall or (vertical) surface. The lights are placed low (usually on the ground) and shine up. Color acetate sheets, called gels, can be placed over the lights to create lighting of different colors.
- **Pin spot:** Focused beam of light that is used to highlight or accent a particular item, such as the cake or the centerpiece at each table.
- **Gobos:** A metal template with a design cut into it that is placed over theatrical or event lighting to produce a pattern on the wall, floor, etc.
- **Spotlight:** A focused beam of light used to draw attention to a particular aspect of the reception such as the entertainment.

If professional event lighting is out of your budget, consider the following:

- **Utilize the venue's lighting system by asking the event manager or your wedding planner to raise and lower the venue's lights at appropriate moments.** Raise the lights during dinner so guests can see, but bring them back down during dancing—nothing can kill the dancing more than a room full of bright lights.
- **Twinkle lights can easily be strung around many railings and trees.** Just be sure to ask your venue if this is okay, allow yourself enough time to do it, and don't forget about extension cords.

On a final note, keep in mind that depending on your venue, you may need to consider utilitarian lighting. Many unique and outdoor venues available to couples do not have the necessary built-in lighting to allow the guests, caterers, and vendors to see properly. You may find yourself in need of lighting services just to pull off the event.

Lighting Checklist

Some areas you may want to highlight with event lighting include:

- ○ Altar/Arch/Location of vows
- ○ Cake table
- ○ Dance floor
- ○ Entrance to the venue/venues
- ○ First dance, spotlight
- ○ Landscape (paths, perimeter of a lawn, a terrace)
- ○ Reception/Guest tables
- ○ Walls (color wash with uplighting)

CHAPTER 14

Ready for My Close-Up

Your wedding day will be one of the most important and most photographed days in your life. You want to make sure that all of your important moments are captured so you will always have the opportunity to look back on images of your precious day and smile. Professionally documenting the important moments of your wedding day in photos and on video is essential for every wedding. Beyond the trends and what you typically see in wedding photography is a whole world of new innovations and ways to capture these special moments.

What You Need to Know

Deciding on the style of photography you prefer and finding a professional photographer you like and work well with you are essential in capturing enduring images of your wedding. With all that goes into finding the right photographer for your wedding, you should acquaint yourself with some basic details that will influence the decisions you make. As you review the following information about photography, keep in mind wedding photography is not necessarily a one-size-fits-all scenario. There are a host of photographers who mix all of these approaches to create their own unique style.

What to Consider

To truly make an informed decision, you need to know that traditional photography is not vegan. Gelatin is used in the production of real film—all film, from x-rays to Hollywood productions to the photos of your wedding day. Not only is gelatin used in the production of the film, it is also used in some of the glossy coatings used during the printing process. Leaving the true vegan option to be digital photos processed with a matte finish.

FACT

Some vegans will shoot with real film, but only when purchased secondhand or if the film is expired, and would otherwise be thrown away. They justify this because it is green and they are reusing someone's castoffs rather than the film clogging up the landfills.

Here is a brief description of some basics you will want to consider as you look at your photography choices.

- **Socially conscious beliefs/green photography.** While this has little to nothing to do with the quality or ability of a photographer, it may be something you really want to consider. Ask yourself the following: Is finding a vegan photographer important to you? Is it important that the photographer is environmentally conscious and utilizes green practices?

- **Photographic style.** Do you want a more photojournalistic approach, which documents the day as it unfolds, with less posing and more spontaneity? Do you prefer a more traditional style of photography that includes more poses, utilizes lighting, and sets up shots? Or does an editorial approach, so that it almost seems as though you are posing for a magazine spread, appeal to you? Once you begin looking at photographers' sample books, your eye will guide you to the style you prefer.

- **Digital or film.** While film was once highly preferred, high-end digital equipment can provide nearly the same quality. Some couples love the look of film, and some want the flexibility of digital. Each type of photography has pros and cons, and ultimately you should not count out either style until you find the photographer you want to hire. In fact, many photographers shoot both formats, and as technology develops, more and more are switching to digital.

- **Black and white or color.** Many couples feel that black-and-white photography has an artistic and timeless appeal. If you are shooting film, it is best to determine this in advance, as some quality may be lost when converting color prints to black and white. With digital, this is not a concern. Even if you love black and white, do not rule out having some color photographs taken. If you like the look of both, ask your photographer if he has the ability to shoot both color and black and white. Shooting with digital opens up new worlds—almost anything is possible.

- **Album selection.** Leather and silk are very popular in the wedding market when it comes time to purchase a wedding album. As a vegan, neither of these options is acceptable to you. Be sure to ask the photographer about other options.

- **Personality.** Beyond the technical and stylistic decision you will make, one important aspect of wedding photography is the rapport you and the photographer have. You should like the photographer you hire. No, he doesn't have to become your new best friend, but his personality should be pleasing to you as well as the manner in which he presents himself. He will be with you much of the day, and he should be someone you feel comfortable with.

Making the Decision

It is of the utmost importance to hire a reliable professional photographer for your wedding. Just imagine how heartbroken you'd be to find that the supposedly professional photographer you hired could only produce blurry, muddy photos, or worse yet, showed up two hours late! It may sound absurd, but such nightmares do happen. Don't let yourself become another victim.

Choose your photographer carefully; only sign on with someone after you've seen his or her work and checked references. It's always wise to interview more than one photographer. That way, you can compare quality and prices to get the best person (and the best deal) for you.

Vegan Values

If strictly adhering to vegan beliefs is important to you, or if being green is, you may also want to ask the following questions:

❍ Are you vegan?
❍ Do you understand what vegan means (obviously, for those not vegan)?
❍ Will you refrain from wearing or bringing any equipment that is obviously derived from animals, such as leather? (Will you keep the leather shoes at home?)
❍ How do you process your prints? Will we be given the option of matte processing?
❍ What album choices do you provide? Do you have options besides silk and leather?
❍ Would you consider yourself to be a green photographer? Why? How?

Questions to Ask

Here is a list of questions that will help you choose the best man, woman, or studio for the job. Some of these questions pertain to film and digital options. As already discussed, digital is the best option for vegans, but some still choose film.

❍ How long has the photographer been in this business?
❍ Does the photographer specialize in weddings (if not a wedding expert, find someone who is)?

○ Is this a full-time photographer?

○ Who is available/will be shooting my wedding (if photographer is part of a larger photography studio)?

○ Does the photographer shoot with a digital camera or with film? Or with both? (Is that acceptable to you?)

○ Does the photographer shoot color only or is black and white or sepia available?

○ Can we see samples of previous work and speak to some former clients?

○ What is the photographer's style?

○ Does the photographer have an assistant? Does the photographer have additional photographers that can be hired to shoot on the wedding day as well?

○ Does the photographer offer an engagement session? At what cost?

○ What types of photo packages are offered?

○ What is included in the standard package?

○ What are the costs for additional photos?

○ How many pictures does the photographer typically take at a wedding of this size?

○ Will we be charged by the hour?

○ Are there travel fees for shooting at more than one location? If the location is over a certain amount of miles from the studio?

○ Does the photographer keep negatives? If so, for how long? If digital, can a disk of all the images be purchased or is it included?

○ May we purchase negatives if we wish (if shot on film)?

○ Will we be able to purchase extra photos in the future?

○ Will the photographer take a mixture of formal and candid shots?

○ Does the photographer shoot bridal portraits?

○ Would the photographer be willing to incorporate our ideas into the shot list?

○ Will the photographer provide a contract stipulating services, date, time, costs, and so on?

○ How long do we have to wait to see the proofs of our wedding photos?

○ How long do we have to wait to receive our albums and final prints of the wedding photos?

Photo Needs

While budget is a concern, when it comes to photography, most couples are first concerned with the style of photography. Most couples want a photographer whose artistic style matches their own.

Most couples prefer to have a combination of posed shots and candid photos. That way they are sure to get as many memories captured on film as possible. Check out the photographer's portfolio to determine what kind of photos she is capable of taking. If you see nothing but posed shots, that's a sign you won't get many candid shots of your wedding.

Once you decide on a photographer, sit down with him to talk about the type and amount of photographs you'd like to see from your wedding. Most professional wedding photographers know what photos they need to take and what photos a bride expects. Ask if he has a standard checklist that he follows for capturing photos. If he doesn't, create one of your own. If he does, check to make sure it includes all the photos you want; add anything that is missing.

ALERT

Even if you are not inclined to request a lot of posed formal portraits, be sure to get shots of your immediate family and any older or special family members or friends. You will treasure these one day.

Traditional Issues and the Digital Age

Now that you have the basic scoop on wedding photography and realize traditional photography is not vegan, it is time to dig deeper into photography and its practices. Photographs may be an important part of human history, a way of remembering and preserving, of creating and envisioning, but some of the basics of photography are not environmentally friendly or vegan. However, our photographs tell a story, and how tragic it would be not to have these parts of our lives documented.

Many of the chemicals used to develop photos are toxic, most photo paper is not recyclable, and the amount of resources and energy that go into making and powering cameras, batteries, lighting, and all the other equipment can be tremendous.

Chemicals 'R Us

As you now know, traditional photography is not vegan, but it is also not eco-friendly. Some of the highly toxic chemicals that are used in the developing process include silver and silver nitrate, diaminophenol hydrochloride, ethylene diamine, formaldehyde, iodine, lead oxalate, hydroquinone, mercuric chloride, acetic acid, ammonium hydroxide, and bromine. These chemicals can cause damage through inhalation or contact with skin. If they are not properly disposed of, they end up in landfills and sewage systems, contaminating soil and groundwater.

The good news for photographers who still process in darkrooms is that there are now safer chemicals such as Kodak's Xtol, one of several new ascorbate (vitamin C) developers. ECO PRO (*www.greenphotochemistry .com*) has several nontoxic solutions.

The Digital Age

Digital technology has made photography an art that is readily accessible to almost everyone while remaining vegan and eco-friendly. There is no need for hazardous chemicals and darkrooms to develop photos. The digital age has made it easier than ever to take, process, and edit photos. Make sure your wedding photographer is on the same green page as you by offering digital proofs and online viewing and ordering. Make sure nothing gets printed except what you specifically choose.

Before digital technology made digital proofs a reality, every single photo was printed out for the couple to view and pick from. The bare minimum number of photos a wedding photographer takes at a wedding is around 500. Most photographers take well over 1,000 photos per wedding. If a couple decided not to purchase their proofs, all those photographs were dumped in the garbage.

Guest Shooter

In addition to hiring a fabulous photographer for your great vegan wedding, get friends and family involved to make sure every aspect of your big day is captured for you to remember. Remind everyone to bring along their cameras. Encourage tech-savvy friends to get creative with photos and prints. Have some switch to black and white or sepia camera settings to get interesting and dramatic photos of your wedding day.

If you want the convenience of single-use cameras at your wedding, consider a camera rental service such as CameraRenter (*www.camerarenter .com*). You choose how many digital cameras you would like to rent, and they come in the mail. Guests take photos with the cameras on your big day then you send the cameras back. CameraRenter creates a custom website with all your photos and videos for easy viewing, sharing, downloading, and print ordering. It also offers options such as custom-created movie DVDs of your event.

ALERT

Disposable cameras produce quite a bit of waste. Even though manufacturers claim that almost all the parts are recyclable, the majority of the cameras still end up in landfills. You also have to develop every single camera, and you have no way of knowing whether the photos are actually good until you have them developed.

What to Do with Digital Photos

Digital technology, combined with the resources of the Internet, has created the opportunity for anyone to become a photo artist. Anyone can create spectacular photo albums, books, and custom-printed materials that once only professionals with expensive equipment and know-how could make. After the wedding, the photos can be e-mailed to you or uploaded to photo-sharing sites, where you can easily share, e-mail, and edit these photos.

Add the photos to your own personal websites and only print the ones you really like. You can even create beautiful photo albums, collages, and many other custom photo keepsakes and gifts. Don't forget to create back-ups of all your photos on CDs or DVDs. Make a copy that can slide right into your wedding keepsake album so it doesn't get lost in the pile of other photo disks.

Greener Photography

Photographers who say they are green or that they offer green photo packages mean they use only digital photo processes. They shoot with digital cameras, and they offer all photos to be proofed digitally. They only print what is requested. This means they are eliminating the use of regular film and the harmful chemicals that are used to develop it. They also cut out paper waste by giving you digital proofs.

Some people will argue that most photographers use digital technology now but they don't label themselves as being green. Digital photographers are quick to label themselves as being green to get a piece of the big eco-pie, but practicing green photography means a lot more than just a digital camera and digitally stored photos.

The Green Photographer

There are many ways photographers can green their business and their lives. Each will have his own passions and his own ways of being as green as he can be. Many may see that becoming green and offering a green wedding package was a natural progression in their lives since they already use digital photo technology, work at home, recycle, and purchase locally grown and organic food.

Many photographers and other business owners take being green very personally, and strive to live a more meaningful, responsible lifestyle. They recycle all paper, packaging, and ink cartridges. They reduce and reuse, and they pass along their beliefs and strive to inspire others.

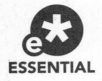

Being green and being a vegan are mindsets that seem to go hand in hand. So when you cannot find a vegan vendor, look for a green vendor. They represent the photographers who are changing their thinking, changing their practices, and therefore changing the world to make it a better place for us all.

Caught on Film

For many couples, live action footage of their wedding is as equally important as the photographic images. How else are the bride and groom going to see and hear everything they were too excited or too dazed to be aware of while it was actually happening? Most couples consider their wedding footage to be priceless so, as with still photography, you should be very careful about whom you choose to trust with the responsibility of capturing your wedding memories as they unfold.

Videography Know-How

With the special moments of your wedding being something that cannot be duplicated, it's usually not a wise idea to hire a family member or friend to be your videographer, even if they do have a shiny new camera. They may do adequate work, but odds are they still can't provide you with the same quality you'll get from a professional. (They probably won't have the necessary editing equipment, for one thing.)

Just as with photography, real film is not vegan, and is produced with the use of gelatin. Luckily, many videographers are making the switch to digital, giving you many more options when it comes time to find the right person to capture the memories of your wedding.

With all of the equipment and technology available today, you should settle for nothing less than a broadcast-quality wedding movie. Get the best deal for your money, but don't choose someone cheap and incompetent over someone who'll cost a little more but do a wonderful job. Just so you know, while it is still called videography, just about all professionals now supply the bride and groom with DVDs, not videotape.

Questions to Ask

When interviewing videographers, heed much of the same advice as when you selected a photographer. For the most part, the same types of questions are applicable and you should apply the same scrutiny. Your videographer will be interacting with you and your guests throughout the wedding, so his personality and his rapport with you and your groom is of the utmost importance. Here are some things you'll want to ask your videographer.

○ How long have you been doing this professionally?
○ Can we see samples of your work and check references?
○ Is the work guaranteed?
○ Do you shoot digitally or on film? Do we have a choice?
○ Can we look at a work in progress in addition to a demo DVD? (This way you'll know that the videographer is actually doing the work, not buying great demo DVDs from someone else.)
○ Is the equipment high quality?
○ How many cameras will be used? How big will the videographer's staff be?
○ What special effects are available?
○ Will you use wireless microphones during the ceremony?
○ How is the fee computed? Flat rate? Hourly?
○ Is a standard package deal offered? Is so, what is it?
○ How much will it cost to have copies of the original made?
○ Is the raw (unedited) footage available for purchase?

WHEN VIEWING SAMPLE DVDS, CONSIDER THE FOLLOWING QUESTIONS:
○ Do the segments tell a story, giving a clear sense of the order in which the events took place?
○ Does the DVD capture the most important moments, such as cutting the cake and throwing the garter?
○ Is there steady use of the camera, clear sound, vibrant color, and a nice sharp picture?
○ How are the shots framed? What editing techniques are used?
○ Does the tape move smoothly from one scene to the next, rather than lurching ahead unexpectedly?

On a final note, be sure to ask your videographer about any new technological advances in cameras or editing that you might be able to take advantage of. Because technology develops so fast, there may be equipment available now that was unheard of even six months ago.

Bridal Beauty and "Groom"ing

With all this talk of preserving these images and memories of the day, of course you want to look your best on your wedding day. And guess what? Your groom probably does, too! Some simple dos and don'ts will assist you with looking your wedding-best!

Hair, Beautiful Hair!

As a bride, you have choices. You can do your hair yourself, or you can hire someone to do it for you—live it up, you are the bride! Depending on who you select to do your hair on the wedding day, you may have to go to the salon or you can find a stylist to come to the comfort and convenience of your home or hotel. Whatever option you choose, take heed of some basic hair dos.

HAIR DOS

- Make an appointment to consult with your hairdresser or hired stylist a few months prior to the wedding.
- Schedule a trial run. Bring your headpiece and ask the stylist to try a few different styling options.
- Ask the hairdresser if you have to make the trek to the salon or if he/she would be able to come to you. How much extra would this cost? Do you have to pay more for work that runs overtime, and how much?
- Make sure the hairdresser knows exactly where and when to meet you.
- Wear a button-down shirt when getting your hair styled. There's nothing worse than suddenly realizing you're going to have to cut yourself out of your favorite shirt, or ruin your hair pulling your shirt over your head.

Put on a Happy Face

Like your hairdresser, a professional makeup artist can help you feel more confident in your appearance, or give you a completely new look. Even if you're already satisfied with your daily makeup selection and application skills, you may want to try something different, something special for your wedding day. A professional makeup artist will ensure you have that wedding day glow without looking overly made up or overdone. On your wedding day it is important that you look and feel comfortable in your own skin. Ultimately, you want to look like a more glamorous version of yourself.

ALERT

Be sure to confirm and reconfirm that the makeup products being used are cruelty free. It may be that the makeup artist never even thought about that. If you are hiring a professional, consider offering her your makeup to use or purchasing new makeup for the wedding day.

MAKEUP DOS

- Schedule a consultation with a trusted makeup artist in your price range.
- Go in for a practice session, just so there are no surprises come the wedding day.
- If you like the makeup application, make an appointment for the day of your wedding.
- Ask if the makeup artist can do your makeup at your home. If yes, how much would this service cost?

Nails

Even if you've always considered manicures to be frivolous, you might want to make an exception for your wedding day. Well-manicured nails and beautiful hands are just another part of the complete bridal beauty package. If your regular routine includes caring for your nails, and that is your preferred look, then you shouldn't need any special attention—just make an appointment with your emery board!

Natural and Organic Beauty Products

There are already many cosmetic companies that create all-natural, safe, organic alternatives. Cruelty-free beauty products can be found in national retailers and drugstores as well as on the web. Drugstore.com and Beauty.com sell several brands of organic and all-natural personal-care products.

Many mainstream companies are adding green cosmetic products to their existing lineups. As a vegan, you want all the products you use to not utilize animal testing or have animal by-products, but you may also be concerned about the use of certified organic ingredients, harsh chemicals, parabens, and synthetic preservatives. Whether or not it comes in recyclable paper containers may also be of concern to you. Look for an ECOCERT certified line of organic makeup.

Look for other companies that support eco-issues. Check to see if companies have signed the Compact for Safe Cosmetics, pledging that their products are free of any potentially harmful chemicals that are known to cause or are suspected of causing cancer or birth defects. You can find these companies through *www.safecosmetics.org*.

DIY Beauty

You can even make your own natural beauty products with many ingredients you may already have in your kitchen: sea salt, cornstarch, cornmeal, honey, oatmeal, sugar, and many fresh fruits, vegetables, and herbs. Food oils that are used as bases for many natural beauty products include almond, apricot kernel, avocado, castor, coconut, jojoba bean, macadamia nut, olive, sesame, soybean, sunflower seed, and wheat germ oils. These natural oils are safe alternatives to chemical-laden body lotions, creams, and oils. A good rule of thumb is, if you wouldn't put it in your body, you shouldn't put it on your body.

CHAPTER 15

The Time of Your Life

Many brides feel pressured to have a large, formal reception because they think their guests expect it, or, more often than not, because it is what brides think a wedding reception is supposed to be. A modern wedding honors tradition, but reinvents itself to suit the bride and groom, so that at the end of the day everyone has celebrated and enjoyed themselves and the couple has stayed true to their beliefs and personalities. So dance the night away, and enjoy this once-in-a-lifetime feeling!

The Perfect Party

While the marriage is truly the most important aspect of the day, many brides spend much time (sometimes too much) planning the reception. Though it is fun, it can also be stressful, as many brides feel pressured to live up to a certain standard. Truth is, the guests just want to celebrate with you, and a reception can be just about anything you want it to be. Deciding between an informal cocktail hour or a plated meal is only part of the story; there is more to the reception than just the meal.

What Happens When

The wedding reception is most likely the biggest and most expensive party you will ever plan. It is the ultimate celebration of this glorious event in your life. After the many, many months you have been planning and looking forward to this day, it is time to relax and enjoy the fruits of your labor with your family and friends.

A wedding reception has three basic parts to it: the cocktail hour, meal service, and dancing. Below are brief explanations of each:

- **The cocktail hour lasts for approximately one hour (sometimes a little less, sometimes a little more).** It allows the couple and wedding party to finish up with their photos and freshen up before the grand entrance. Now, if you feel uncomfortable calling this cocktail hour—because of the time of day or even due to religious considerations—feel free to simply call this a gathering time.
- **At the conclusion of the cocktail hour, the guests are escorted to the dining area for the meal.** Once they find their seats, the first order of business is the grand entrance. Then your wedding meal will be served. Traditional elements will continue throughout the meal and remainder of the evening.
- **Once the meal is complete, dancing begins and the party really starts.** More than likely, there will be formal protocol dancing and then the guests will be invited to join in. The cake is cut, and the bouquet and garter are tossed.

Traditions

There are many ways to structure the flow of events at a wedding reception. It really just depends on what you want to do and what kind of reception you want to have. You can work with your wedding planner, location manager, and musical entertainment to personalize or develop your itinerary. Use the following list to assist you with determining which traditions you may or may not want to include in your own reception timeline.

ESSENTIAL

While veganism is not a tradition, it is an integral part of your life, and if at some point you choose to make a note of the vegan values, hey, it's your wedding. Just do it tactfully and don't preach. Consider a small note on your menu card that refers to the vegan menu.

Keep in mind what all these traditions mean and what they are for as you prepare the reception timeline in this chapter. At that time, you will be formulating the specific details of these events as well as selecting appropriate musical selections to accompany them.

RECEPTION TRADITIONS AND EVENTS CHECKLIST

○ **Grand entrance of couple:** The grand entrance is the first introduction of the bride and groom at the reception. This is generally the first order of business once the guests are in their seats, as everyone's attention is focused. Traditionally, the bride and groom as well as the entire wedding party are formally announced into the reception, but recently, couples are making a change and only introducing the bride and groom.

○ **Welcome by bride's father:** This is an optional activity. If you choose to include it, the father of the bride (or host of the wedding) usually greets and welcomes the guests soon after the guests take their seats, prior to the best man's toast.

○ **Toast by best man:** The best man traditionally makes the first toast. His toast should take place toward the beginning of the evening—following the grand entrance or before or after the first course is served. It is quite common for the maid of honor to have her turn at the microphone. Her toast should follow the best man's.

○ **Bride and groom greet guests:** This is a popular option in lieu of having a receiving line. During the meal service (once you have eaten), the bride and groom go from table to table to greet the guests.

○ **First dance:** Traditionally, no one should take the dance floor until the bride and groom have danced their first dance. There are many opportunities to do the first dance earlier in the reception so that if your guests are feeling the music and want to get up and dance, the floor will be open. A very popular option is to do the first dance immediately following the grand entrance; as the bride and groom enter the venue, they go directly to the dance floor and right into their dance. It may also be done between courses or as the meal concludes.

○ **The father/daughter dance:** This is the second dance of the evening, but it doesn't necessarily need to immediately follow the first dance. For example, if the first dance followed the grand entrance, the father/daughter dance can be held after the first course is served or once the meal concludes. This is followed by the mother/son dance.

○ **Wedding-party dance:** The wedding-party dance is purely optional to begin with, so you may choose to skip it. If you do want to have a wedding-party dance, each attendant can dance with their spouse/significant other, matching up those who are not married with other members of the wedding party.

○ **Cake cutting:** The cake cutting is a lovely tradition that can quickly turn ugly. Everyone has seen the images of a bride and groom smashing cake into each other's faces. Really, no one wants to walk around with cake up their nose. So, take the dignified route. Make a pact to have a classy and sweet cake cutting that the guests will remember for all the right reasons. The bride and groom cut the first piece of cake together. A small slice of cake is placed on a plate, and then the groom feeds the bride a small bite, followed by the bride doing the same to the groom. Cake is then served to the guests.

- ○ **Bride and groom toast/thank you speech:** At some point during the reception, the groom toasts the bride, the bride toasts the groom, or the couple thanks the guests for coming.
- ○ **Garter and bouquet toss:** The long-standing tradition of these events is that whoever catches the bouquet or garter will be the next to marry. This typically calls for the single men/ladies at the reception to gather in a particular area so that the bride/groom may (blindly) toss the garter/bouquet. If you are planning to do the toss, ask the florist to make you a toss bouquet; these are usually included at little to no charge. Keep in mind, you are not required to do either of these, or you can just do one or the other.
- ○ **Send off or getaway:** It is the formal exit of the newlyweds, and the conclusion of the event. One way to do this is to have guests line a path, and the bride and groom make their way through the guests to their transportation and are whisked away. Depending on the rules of the venue, guests may shower the couple with rose petals, bubbles, or light sparklers. Another option is to have the emcee play a last-dance song, and gather the guests on the dance floor. At some point toward the middle to end of the song, the emcee cues you to exit and the guests are left to finish the dance while you head out.

Setting the Mood

From the moment guests arrive to the last dance, the music tells the story of the day, and a lot about the two of you. By selecting varied styles of music, everyone will find something to keep them entertained. Whether you select traditional secular music or folk music or a good old rock 'n' roll tune, it is your day to express yourself through your love and the music you select.

Location Connection

Before you begin interviewing musical entertainment, you may need to discuss the following items with your location manager. It would be heart-breaking for you to shell out thousand of dollars on a band to later discover that your venue is located in a residential area and amplified music is not allowed, or that your rural locale has no power. Additionally, you may want to visit the site with your band or disc jockey before making any formal commitment.

- ❍ Can the reception site accommodate your band or disc jockey?
- ❍ Is there enough electrical power? Outlets? Space?
- ❍ How are the acoustics?
- ❍ Are there restrictions on amplified sound or a noise curfew at the venue?

Who Ya Gonna Call?

Carefully selected music can provide atmosphere and enhance the mood and meaning of your special day. You may already have an auditory fantasy of the music that will be playing as you walk down the aisle, as you take your vows, leave the church, and dance your first dance as husband and wife . . . but who's going to play it? Quality musicians and bands as well as disc jockeys provide the key to fulfilling the experience and completing the picture-perfect memory of your wedding day.

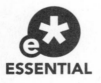

ESSENTIAL

Search the web to find vegan and like-minded musicians in your area. Try checking local vegan groups. Ask your friends—don't count out the results a post on some social networking sites could yield—you never know where that great vegan band is hiding!

Vegan Considerations

When it comes time to select your musicians, you may encounter an obstacle or two, other than the guitarist showing up in leather pants. Many instruments contain animal products. For example, the glue on wooden instruments is derived from animals, and the bow of the violin is typically made from horse hair, and drums generally include some variety of animal hide.

Depending on where you live and the abundance of vegan musicians in the area, your decision may be greatly influenced by these factors. There are vegan alternatives to these issues, but unless your musicians are vegan they may or may not have access to or care to use alternatives.

ESSENTIAL

What are you going to do if you find "the" band, but the instruments are not necessarily vegan? Go with your gut feeling and realize sometimes it is just not possible to exclude all animal products when you have no control over the source. Does this preclude you from listening to major bands or classical music every day?

Church Musicians

Before you hire a full orchestra to accompany the church choir, though, remember that the cost of musicians and singers for the ceremony must fit into your overall music budget. In other words, you don't hire a $1,000 string quartet when you have only $1,200 allotted for ceremony and reception music. It may take some fancy footwork, but don't be intimidated. You can have wonderful music for both events with a little compromise and ingenuity.

Most churches have musicians available for you to hire at a very reasonable price. Some will allow you to bring in your own musicians, provided they meet the church's guidelines. In other words, unless you belong to a very progressive church, your favorite local hard-rock band probably won't be allowed to set up in the choir loft.

If your friends are no help and your church doesn't have a wedding coordinator, you'll have to hit the wedding circuit in town. Sit through some weddings—if you hear a great soloist, grab him or her after the ceremony and make arrangements to meet and discuss your wedding.

You may even ask the music department at your local high school or community college if there are any students who sing (or play the trumpet, piano, violin) at weddings. Seek out the director of the music program at a local college. Look in the classified section of your newspaper. The musicians are out there—you just have to hunt them down.

Who Will Rock Your Reception?

The size, formality, and budget of your wedding should help determine the type of entertainment you have at the reception. At a very formal affair, there may be a strolling violinist or a piano player who will provide background music as the meal is served. If you're having your reception in a private home or a backyard, you can play your own CDs and pipe them through a good stereo system. That will provide plenty of music to dance to.

Once you decide on the kind of music you want at your wedding, you need to find someone to provide it. You may already have someone in mind, like the disc jockey who played at your cousin's wedding or your favorite local vegan band. If you don't have a clue, ask friends, relatives, and coworkers. Perhaps they've been to or hosted a wedding recently and can recommend—or steer you away from—a certain band or disc jockey.

These days, the big musical decision is whether to hire a band or a disc jockey. When it comes to price, the disc jockey is definitely the less expensive option, but there are other factors that may influence your choice. Whichever you select, you will want to finalize arrangements approximately six months in advance of your wedding date.

Live Versus Recorded

Depending on whom you talk to, you will hear many arguments about why a disc jockey is better than a band or vice versa. Ultimately, it comes down to the couple's preference for prerecorded music versus live music. Bands look impressive up on the stage, and have traditionally been considered more formal than disc jockeys. However, bands are considerably more expensive than disc jockeys, and many couples want to hear their musical selections as they know them, not as a band plays them, so either choice has become perfectly acceptable at a formal wedding. The disc jockey or bandleader also typically acts as emcee for the event.

When you are selecting the musical entertainment, there is no reason you have to settle for a loud band or a cheesy disc jockey that will spoil the mood. Professionals will tailor their repertoire to your needs. When you interview a band or disc jockey tell them what you are expecting and if they cannot or will not do it, look elsewhere.

Disc Jockeys

Disc jockeys are fast becoming the wedding music option of choice. Disc jockeys can provide more variety than a band. They give you the original version of a song, and they're less of a logistical headache. Disc jockeys are seen as slightly less formal than bands, but they're also considerably less expensive, which adds a great deal to their appeal.

It's just as important to see and hear a disc jockey in action as it is with a band. Look for the same things you would in a band: balance, variety, a good mix of fast and slow songs, a good personality, and first-rate equipment. Could this person perform the duties of master of ceremonies? Does he talk way too much or far too little?

Live Bands

Assuming you can find a charismatic, golden-throated singer backed by talented, enthusiastic musicians, there is no substitute for a live band. If you're lucky enough to find live musicians who can work within your budget, snap them up quickly—before another bride hires your band for her wedding.

ALERT

Just to cover your bases, if you hire a rockin' rock 'n' roll band, double check what their typical attire is. Leather is almost a staple for rockers. Ask if they can leave the leather at home, and if they agree, get it in the contract . . . that includes their guitar straps!

In addition to the band's sound, look for a variety of musical styles and tempos in their repertoire. Do they play seven slow songs, one fast number, then two more slow ones, or do they know how to vary the pace? Do they appear to be enjoying themselves, or do they look like they'd rather be somewhere else?

It's a Deal

Once you find a band you like, make arrangements with the leader to sit down and talk about exactly what you want from the band concerning your wedding. Have a list of songs ready that you have to hear at your reception. If they don't know the songs already, will they attempt to learn them in time? Ask about their sound system and equipment needs. If your reception site is too small, or doesn't have the proper electrical outlets and fuse power, it's better to know before you hire the band.

FACT

At most weddings, the bandleader or disc jockey doubles as the master of ceremonies. If you want your bandleader to perform this duty, find out whether he or she will be willing and if any extra cost is involved.

Make sure whoever will be acting as emcee has the poise and charisma to handle the responsibility. You don't want the microphone in the hands of someone who will insult your guests, make jokes as you cut the cake, or mumble your names unintelligibly as you enter the reception site for the first time as husband and wife!

Questions to Ask

As with every wedding vendor you hire, you should interview the musicians carefully and ask for references. Use the following questions when interviewing potential entertainers.

- ❍ What is the band's specialty?
- ❍ Do you specialize in rock 'n' roll, jazz, blues, etc.? (For a DJ) Do you specialize in a certain style or sound or genre of music?
- ❍ How many members are in the band? (For a DJ) Do you work alone or do you have an assistant?
- ❍ What equipment do you bring? Do you have a song list we must select from? Are you willing to learn/find special requests?
- ❍ What are the fees? How many hours does that include? Is overtime available? At what cost?
- ❍ How many breaks do you require during a typical four- or five-hour reception? How do you accommodate our musical needs during your breaks?
- ❍ What are the costs?
- ❍ Are there any added fees not included in the quote?
- ❍ Will the disc jockey's/band's attire be appropriate for the reception?
- ❍ Is a special sound system or hookup required?
- ❍ What is the cancellation policy?
- ❍ What are the payment terms? (Ask about deposit and balance amounts.)
- ❍ What are the hourly overtime rates?
- ❍ If songs that are important to us are not currently in the repertoire or play list, can they be added? Is there any additional charge for this?

Hiring the Band

Before you sign a contract with the band, make sure the following commitments are stipulated in writing:

○ The band's attire. You don't want them showing up at a formal wedding in ripped jeans and gym shorts. Or at your vegan wedding in leather pants!

○ The band's arrival time. Make sure the band is set up, with instruments tuned, before the guests arrive. The band's sound check will probably not make for soothing dinner music.

○ The exact cost of hiring the band and everything included for that price. Some bands charge you if they have to add an extra piece of equipment; others charge a fee for playing requests.

This is also the time to make sure the band knows the exact location of the reception. There have actually been instances where the musical talent has shown up at the reception site with the right name but in the wrong city.

Hiring the Disc Jockey

Find out how big his music collection is, as your disc jockey should be able to accommodate the majority of your guests' requests. Provide a list of what you want played at the reception, and if you have some songs you absolutely, positively, upon penalty of death do not want played, give him a hit list of those, too! If some of the music you want isn't available, is the DJ willing to purchase it? Some other questions to ask your DJ include:

○ How many weddings has he provided music for? What size weddings does he typically work?

○ Will he provide appropriate music for the cocktail hour?

○ Does he provide a wireless microphone for any toasts or speeches?

○ Is gratuity included in the price?

The DJ's exact cost, including possible extras, the time of arrival and departure, the place, and his proper attire should all be spelled out in the contract that you sign.

Here Comes the Bride

Before you begin to pick out music for your wedding ceremony, keep in mind that in a house of worship, the music will most likely need to be religious in tone. Be sure to check with the officiant or your house of worship for current guidelines, as policies on what selections are appropriate in a religious setting do evolve. It's a good idea to find out what you can and can't use before you get your heart set on something. On the other hand, if your wedding is not being held in a house of worship, almost anything goes.

You should also:

○ Meet with the musical director from your house of worship to discuss appropriate selections.
○ Discuss fees for the organist and any additional musicians that may be provided.
○ Begin to choose the selection for each distinct part of the ceremony at least two months before the wedding.

The Prelude

The prelude music sets the mood, and provides some listening enjoyment for your guests while they await your arrival. It should begin twenty to thirty minutes prior to the ceremony start time, and come to an end as the mothers and grandmothers are preparing to be escorted down the aisle.

The Processional

After the mothers are seated, the processional is played as the wedding party makes its way down the aisle. When the bride begins her walk, something selected especially for her is played. (An alternative, however, is for the bride to walk down the aisle to the same tune as the rest of the party, played at a different tempo.)

The Ceremony

During the ceremony itself, you may wish to hear songs that have a special meaning for you and your groom. It is very nice to have a piece of music played while the couple is participating in symbolic rituals where there is no speaking, such as the lighting of the unity candle, the wine ceremony, or taking communion. If nothing comes to mind, ask your officiant for ideas. She will probably be able to suggest dozens of wonderful songs that can add meaning to what's taking place.

The Recessional

The recessional is played at the conclusion of the ceremony, as the members of the wedding party make their way back down the aisle. This music should be joyous and upbeat to reflect the new happiness in your life. Many couples are making a break from the traditional and playing modern musical selections that really reflect their personalities. Of course, if you are in a house of worship, be sure to check if you can play modern tunes for the recessional.

Cocktails, Anyone?

There are many ways to go about choosing your cocktail music; what is important is that the music has general appeal, is pleasing to listen to, and not loud or overwhelming so that people cannot converse. The cocktail hour is the time when the wedding party and families finish with the photography and the guests arrive at the reception location. During this time, refreshments and light fare should be served.

Entertaining Options

Along with serving refreshments, it is a nice touch to provide some entertainment to keep the guests happy and the overall good feel of the wedding moving along.

ENTERTAINMENT OPTIONS
- Prerecorded music from the venue sound system
- An iPod or mp3 player
- Ask the disc jockey if he can provide a small sound system for the cocktail area
- Ask the band if a couple of the musicians are available to play (and then join the band later)

- Hire live musicians—anything from a strolling guitarist to a mini orchestra
- If you are really up for something different, you can hire magicians, fortune tellers, or tarot-card readers

Tuning up the Reception

The music at your reception is a key element in the success of your reception. You will need to select appropriate music that appeals to all ages for a truly successful musical plan. Additionally, you may want to include music and dances from your family's ethnic heritage to liven up your reception.

Reception Details

When you hire professional musical entertainment, you do not need to direct the musical selections for every moment of the reception, as they should be able to read the crowd's mood and, through their experience, judge what music would be appropriate based on prior discussions with you. There will, however, be some events throughout the reception that you will want to select special pieces of music for.

Following is a checklist of events that your master of ceremonies (i.e., band leader, disc jockey, or other) and reception-site coordinator will discuss with you in regards to your reception itinerary. Complete this form to determine the happenings at your reception and include your preferred musical selection for the events. Once you do this, your reception will take shape quickly.

RECEPTION MUSIC CHECKLIST

Introduce entire bridal party? Yes___   No___

Music: _____

Introduce only bride and groom? Yes___ No___

Music: _____

Parent(s) of bride: _____

Parent(s) of groom: _____

Grandparent(s) of bride: _____

Grandparent(s) of groom: _____

Flower girl(s): _____

Ring bearer(s): _____

Bridesmaids:

_____

_____

_____

Groomsmen/Ushers:

_____

_____

_____

Maid/Matron of honor: _____

Best man: _____

Bride and groom as they are to be introduced: _____

_____

Receiving line at reception?   Yes___ No___ When ___

Music: _____

Blessing?   Yes___   No___

By whom: _____

First toast? Yes____   No____

By whom: _____

Other toasts?   Yes____   No____

By whom:

_____

_____

_____

First dance: Yes____   No____   When___

Music: _____

To join in first dance: _____

Maid of honor and best man?   Yes____   No____

Parents of bride and groom?   Yes____   No____

Bridesmaids and ushers? Yes____   No____

Guests?   Yes____   No____

Father/daughter dance? Yes____   No____

Music: _____

Mother/son dance?　　　Yes____　　　No____

Music: _____

Wedding-party dance?　　Yes____　　　No____

Music: _____

Open dance floor for guests after first dance?　　Yes____　　　No____

Cake cutting?　　Yes____　　　No____

Music: _____

Bouquet toss?　　Yes____　　　No____

Music: _____

Garter toss?　　Yes____　　　No____

Music: _____

Last dance?　　Yes____　　　No____

Music: _____

Other event: _____

When: _____

Music: _____

Other event: _____

When: _____

Music: _____

CHAPTER 16

Rehearsals, Guests, and Gifts, Oh My!

They're coming! They're coming! Yes, the guests are finally coming. Now what are you going to do with them? Having people come from all over to attend your wedding is an honor. You can make it a smooth journey for them by providing travel information, activities to entertain them, and a warm welcome to greet them upon their arrival. Don't forget about planning the wedding rehearsal and the rehearsal dinner. The countdown begins!

Let's Practice

You want everything to flow smoothly on your wedding day, and a well-orchestrated rehearsal is the key to success. Usually, the night before the wedding you will gather all involved parties at the ceremony site, so that they can familiarize themselves with the venue and participate in a quick run-through of the ceremony. When all is done, it is off to a fun and relaxing evening with friends and family at the rehearsal dinner.

Why a Rehearsal?

The rehearsal is mainly a chance to show everyone the order of the wedding day's events and prepare them for the ceremony. It also gives the families and wedding party a chance to acquaint themselves with the location.

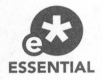

ESSENTIAL

Prepare an itinerary for each member of the wedding party, the family, and other important players on the wedding day. Include arrival times, contact phone numbers, addresses, and other important aspects of their duties as necessary. Pass these copies out to everyone at the rehearsal.

Planning the Rehearsal

The rehearsal is basically to let everyone involved know what to do, where to go, and when to do it. The officiant or wedding planner will do a quick run-through of the ceremony from processional to recessional, making sure that the wedding party and parents know their positions and seats; ushers learn all their duties; readers practice their readings; and soloists run through their pieces. Use this opportunity to point out the bride's room, restrooms, and where photos will be taking place. Finally, the wedding planner or officiant will go over rules or special information.

ALERT

Be sure to ask if the officiant you hired will be attending the rehearsal. You should also clarify if this is included in his fee or if there is an additional charge. If the officiant attends the rehearsal, he and his spouse should be invited to the dinner.

If you are marrying at a house of worship, the wedding coordinator for the location usually runs the rehearsal. At most offsite venues, it is typical for an officiant to not attend the rehearsal, potentially leaving you on your own to rally the troops. If you do not have a wedding planner, you need to be a very organized bride. First, work things out very clearly with your officiant as far as the sequence of events for the ceremony, including how the processional and recessional should be orchestrated. Plan out how you want everyone to enter and where they will stand as well as where you want the parents to be seated. If possible, enlist the help of a friend who is not in the wedding party to assist at the rehearsal. Or better yet, to ease your load, look into hiring a wedding planner to run the rehearsal and the ceremony on the wedding day.

The Rehearsal Dinner

Immediately following the rehearsal is the rehearsal dinner. This is a time for the people involved in the wedding to gather together and enjoy some special, more intimate time together prior to the big day. As far as rehearsal dinners go, they need not be dinners at all; luncheons are perfectly acceptable. The style of menu will be dictated by the time of the wedding rehearsal.

The Vegan Experience

Traditionally, the groom's parents plan and host the rehearsal dinner. You may definitely hear some groans about it being vegan, depending on how accepting and understanding the groom's parents are of the vegan lifestyle. You must take the time to work out a plan and make sure everyone who is involved is willing to play by the rules before rehearsal day. It is too late to have this discussion while the waiters are serving the surf and turf plates at the steak house.

What do you do when you need to make his parents happy but you do not want to go against your own beliefs? Well, just like the marriage, this is a compromise, too. Here are some options:

- If the parents or hosts are not knowledgeable of the vegan life or you think they may be noncompliant in their planning, you may choose to take matters into your own hands and host the rehearsal dinner yourself.
- A frank talk may be in order and make sure you have the groom in on it, since they are his parents. Be kind but firm, and offer up a list of menu ideas as well as vegan condiments, desserts, and organic wines.
- Optional: If you are making compromises on the wedding day by serving an animal protein, either suggest the rehearsal dinner is a completely vegan event due to that fact, or let them make the same menu concessions as the wedding day menu.

Who's Invited?

Strictly speaking, the following people should be invited: immediate families of the couple (parents, siblings, grandparents), the wedding party and their spouses/significant others (not dates) and their children (if they have traveled to attend the wedding), any children in the wedding party and their parents (depending on the time of the dinner), and the officiant and his spouse.

FACT

It is not necessary to invite all the out-of-town guests to the rehearsal dinner. If money and space permit, inviting the out-of-town guests is a nice gesture, but it is not required.

What's It For?

Technically you do not need to have a rehearsal dinner, but it is expected and customary. A rehearsal dinner need not be a dinner, either; it can be a brunch or lunch, whatever coincides with the rehearsal time best. The atmosphere is typically more relaxed and intimate than the wedding, and therefore it is a perfect time for more personal toasts from the wedding party and parents.

ESSENTIAL

A rehearsal dinner should not, in size or formality, eclipse the actual wedding. Watch the size of your guest list and take into account the events of the wedding day. For example, if you are planning a casual barbecue for the wedding, a four-course rehearsal dinner would be out of place.

Traditions

Besides having a good time, there is nothing that is required at the rehearsal dinner. Many times the couple will present the attendants with gifts, and there will be a round of toasts. As for the gifts, they are a small thank you for all the work and money your wedding party has put into the wedding.

It's also nice for you and your fiancé to give gifts to your respective parents. When it is time to toast, the groom can toast his bride and future in-laws, and the bride can toast her groom and future in-laws. Sometimes, the couple's parents like to get in a few words as well. Feel free to have as many toasts as you'd like; if everyone wants to make a toast and the mood calls for it, let them! Try to have these toasts in the intimacy of the rehearsal dinner, rather than at the reception.

Who Pays?

Traditionally, the groom's parents have the honor and expense of hosting the rehearsal dinner. However, it is not a faux pas for the bride's parents to throw the dinner if for some reason the groom's parents cannot. The bride's parents, and even you and your fiancé, can pitch in for the dinner. Whoever is hosting should consult the bride and groom about locations and other details.

QUESTION

Do we need to send formal invitations for the rehearsal dinner?
A phone call can suffice as an invitation, but sending a printed invitation is perfectly fine. The invitations need not be formal, and can simply be purchased at the local stationery store or printed on the computer.

Thank You for Coming

When guests travel near or far to attend your wedding, it is customary and polite to thank them for their attendance and support. There are different ways to do this, from a traditional receiving line to individually greeting them at their tables to presenting them with mementos of the occasion.

The Receiving Line

The receiving line gets a fair amount of bad press, mainly because couples are not quite sure what it entails or what to do. They can only envision a long line of anxious guests waiting . . . and waiting. So, it's usually the first thing to get axed. However, with proper protocol and a plan, the receiving line can be a lot of fun for you, and it is a great way to connect with the guests.

Traditionally, the receiving line should form after the ceremony but before the reception. You can have it at either site. Just keep in mind that the receiving line is only as time consuming as you make it. Here's who may participate (in order, beginning at the head of the line):

- Bride's mother
- Bride's father (optional)
- Groom's mother
- Groom's father (optional)

- Bride
- Groom
- Maid of honor
- Best man (optional)
- Bride's attendants

Traditionally, the fathers' and the best man's participation in the receiving line are optional and not considered to be traditional. If you do choose to include them, their proper positions are outlined above.

In the receiving line, you should welcome your guests, thank them for coming, and introduce them to the other members of the wedding party. If a guest is unknown to you, your groom or someone else in your wedding party may introduce you. Be friendly but brief; otherwise, the line may take too long.

Table Hopping

There is nothing wrong with not having a receiving line, and in fact, skipping it can get the reception started ASAP. It is imperative that you greet your guests and make them feel welcomed. Provided it doesn't interfere with serving the meal, go table to table to greet the guests throughout the event. Continue between courses, during the meal, and if necessary, as the dancing begins. Your parents may also want to visit the tables.

ALERT

Just as you would in a receiving line, make the guest feel special, but keep it short, spending only five minutes or so per table. Otherwise, you will spend your evening visiting tables and doing nothing else.

"Favor"able Ideas

Wedding favors began centuries ago. Rich European aristocrats would show off their wealth by offering opulent gifts to wedding guests. The extravagant gifts were originally small, fancy boxes, known as bonbonnieres in France and bomboniere in Italy. They were often made of porcelain, crystal, or gold and encrusted with precious gemstones. Contained inside the box was a bonbon or other sugary treat. Today, wedding favors are a multimillion dollar industry all by themselves. Go vegan and introduce the guests to a whole new, cruelty-free world.

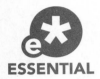

There are vast and varied options for providing amazing favors for your wedding guests. There truly is something for everyone. So take a peek and see what you can handcraft or find in a thrift store. If that is not up your alley, consider some of these great organic ideas, or make a donation to one of your favorite charities. Now, aren't you a lucky bride with all of these options?

Do You Need Them?

Favors aren't necessary, but most couples like to present their guests with a little something. Favors are a tradition, and in recent years have become quite elaborate, but they need not be. Favors make the most sense when they relate to the theme or represent something about the bride and groom. Your budget will ultimately decide the favor. Brides have given something as simple as a packet of seeds and as elaborate as hand-painted scarves for a chilly winter wedding. If you are giving a tasty vegan treat, like a piece of chocolate or cookies, it should be per person. If you are giving something like a picture frame or a candle, one per couple is fine.

What to Give

The wedding favor is an excellent opportunity for you to get some great vegan products into the guests' hands. Exceptional vegan candies, candles, or bath products would make great favors. Tokens inspired by your locale or destination are a fun and meaningful gift as well. Honestly, the possibilities only end with your imagination, but here are some ideas to get you on the right track.

Organic and Edible Favors

Edible favors are always a hit. Chances are food favors won't end up in the garbage; they'll end up in someone's belly. If you have leftovers that no one takes home, they can go home with you or you can donate them to a food bank. There are many organic treats you can give as favors—anything from candy to wine to spiced nuts. Small decorative bottles can be purchased for homemade vinegars, oils, or syrups. If you aren't handy in the kitchen, don't despair! Health food stores and many Internet shops sell organic goodies in bulk that can be used for fabulous favors.

Eco-Favors

Some eco-favors may not be flashy, but they can be extremely practical and therefore very green. Green is all about being useful, particularly when it comes to reusing materials. Give your guests a favor they will use; as a bonus, they will showcase what you and your wedding are all about.

FACT

A CFL (compact fluorescent light) bulb will last six to ten times longer than a regular incandescent light bulb and save at least $45 worth of energy in its lifetime. Australia and other nations have even banned incandescent bulbs altogether. In the United States, manufacturers are selling greater numbers of CFL bulbs.

You could give each guest reusable tote bags, CFL light bulbs, green cleaning supplies, organic bath and body products, organic soaps, or even carbon offset certificates. Rechargeable batteries and battery chargers, mini LED flashlights, a strand of LED lights, or other energy-efficient gifts also make great eco-favors.

You can also consider giving guests organic cotton, hemp, or bamboo washcloths or kitchen towels or kitchen utensils. Including a little brochure (printed on recycled paper, of course) with a list of green-living websites and local stores that offer green products is a thoughtful touch. Depending on the size of your wedding, you might even be able to give gift certificates or coupons to one of the stores. A list of do-it-yourself green cleaning recipes might inspire your guests to think green—and it will make them think of you every time they use it.

Vintage Favors

Little vintage accessories are sweet, charming, and eco-fabulous favors. You might be able to find costume jewelry pieces, hatpins, hairpins or clips, cuff links, tie tacks, buttons, or vintage hankies. Vintage ornaments would be wonderful for a winter wedding around the holidays. Books—especially old poetry books—are a creative choice. Put a custom label on the inside of each book to thank your guests for attending. The books could even be grouped together in the center of the table for an unusual centerpiece. Other vintage favor ideas might be old cosmetic compacts, business card holders, and other small trinkets that are commonly found in antique shops.

ALERT

Search through your old family photo albums for vintage wedding photos. It would be a wonderfully personal touch to incorporate vintage wedding memories from your own family into your big day. Go through the photos with your older relatives, and ask them questions about their own weddings.

Handmade Favors

Making your own favors can be a truly rewarding experience. Imagine walking around your wedding, where everyone is oohing and ahhing all over the fabulous favors, and being able to smile and proudly say, "I made that." Need some quick inspiration for favors you can make yourself? Here's a list of relatively easy-to-make crafts that can be made with cruelty-free products and customized to fit your theme, color scheme, and budget:

- Handmade paper crafts such as note cards or stationery
- All-natural soaps
- Bath salts, bath bombs, scrubs, or oils
- Potpourri
- Scented sachets
- Handcrafted soy candles
- Fire-starter bundles, great for late fall or winter weddings
- Key chains made from found and recycled materials

Charitable Giving

Make your favors really meaningful by purchasing them from charities or from organizations whose proceeds are donated to charities. There are many charitable organizations that you could donate to instead of purchasing favors. Pick something that you are passionate about. This is the perfect opportunity to support charities and causes that you as a vegan believe so strongly in. Animal rights, animal shelters, and conservation organizations are great choices.

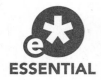

ESSENTIAL

Instead of printing hundreds of favor cards, posting just one big sign is a great way to conserve paper and other resources. Post the sign near the entrance or near your guest book so that everyone will see it. You could also choose to have your emcee announce your donation.

No matter what charity you choose, it is meaningful and it matters. Every little bit counts. You might even want to check your area for local charities and organizations that could use your help. Charity (*www.charity.com*) and JustGive (*www.justgive.org*) are two good online resources to help hook you up with a charity.

Living Gifts

The greenest gifts are those that grow. What better way to share your love for each other and your love for the environment than by giving your guests seeds, trees, or plants they can enjoy for weeks, months, and even years to come? The options for favors that grow are practically as limitless as the multitude of trees, flowers, and seeds you can find.

Considerations

A living gift is a great selection, but before you run out and start purchasing or planting, really think about how feasible this idea is in your area, at your wedding, and during the specific time of the year.

You should consider several things when you choose a live favor:

- Is the plant species native to the area where you and the majority of your guests live?
- When is the optimal time for planting it in the ground? For instance, if you're getting married in October, you might not want to give a tree that should be planted in the spring.
- What is your budget for favors?
- Where will you store all the plants or trees until the wedding, and how easy will it be to transport all of them to the reception location?
- How hardy are the plants? You don't want to buy fragile plants that could perish at any given moment before the wedding.

Living Green Options

If you are up for the task of providing guests with living favors, here are some great ideas that the guests will be sure to love:

- **Small trees, small potted plants, potted flowers, and lucky (curly) bamboo** all make good green favors.
- **Homegrown plants support the grow-your-own food movement.** Give fruit or vegetable plants that grow well in containers such as berries, tomatoes, or peppers. Culinary herbs are rather easy to grow in small

containers, and there are many to choose from, including basil, oregano, thyme, chives, and several kinds of mint.

- **Trees are popular favor options.** They are sometimes harder to start from seed, so you may want to purchase seedlings that are already well established. Tree in a Box (*www.treeinabox.com*) offers many styles for wedding favors and gifts, and the Arbor Day Foundation (*www.arborday.org*) has a wedding package that consists of your choice of redwoods, pines, or spruces. You can make a customized label with a personal message, and the tree comes in a tube that can be converted into a bird feeder.
- **Bulbs are another beautifully green option.** You can give just the bulb itself in a nice little eco-package with directions for planting it, or you can grow bulb flowers in containers or pots.
- **Seeds are a wonderfully green option.** Some companies offer custom-printed seed packets with all your wedding information on them. And there are many companies that offer free printable seed packets that you can customize.

Attendant Gifts

You want your attendant gifts to be bigger and better than the favors you give to everyone else, but you still want them to follow the theme of your wedding. Skip the cookie-cutter attendant gifts such as money clips and engraved business-card holders in favor of more eco-friendly gifts. Besides, no one ever uses the faux-crystal ring holder anyway; why not give something that's both practical and environmentally friendly?

Female attendants might enjoy baskets full of organic pampering. Include bath and body oils, lotions, bath salts, bath bombs, soy candles, vegan chocolates, and organic tea. Give the male attendants gifts made from recycled materials—belts or photo frames made from recycled bicycle tires or chains. Music buffs would love a big bowl made from an old vinyl record.

There are definitely some tried-and-true attendants' gifts. You can put your own spin on any of these by purchasing fair-trade, vegan, artisan, locally made, and organic options. You can give all the attendants' the same thing or customize each gift so you know you're giving each attendant something he will use and enjoy.

CHAPTER 17

Planes, Trains, and Hotel Rooms

You can plan a grand event, but if you forget to make logistical arrangements to get people to and from the ceremony and reception—especially the bride—what's it all for? So, let's face it, talking cars may be a guy thing; talking hotel rooms may seem tedious, but it is all necessary, and if you put some thought and creativity into it, you just might have a little fun and create an experience for yourself and your guests that is magical!

Guest Travel

No matter the size or scope, there will be some sort of travel involved in order to get to and from your wedding. Whether it is a destination wedding in Hawaii with only ten of your closest friends and family or a local wedding for 200, travel is always going to be an integral part of making sure the day goes smoothly.

Transportation

The guests are coming, and they have to get here somehow. You are not required to pay for any portion of the guests' travel arrangements. As an acceptance of your invitation, they assume the responsibility of paying their own way to your wedding. Of course, if your financial situation can accommodate such arrangements, it is perfectly okay to do so.

FACT

Arranging group airfare discounts will provide some welcome economic relief for guests that will be flying in to attend your wedding. Generally, the airlines ask that a minimum number of fares are purchased from them in exchange for a discount. Check out the airline's website or call them directly to find out their requirements.

Providing transportation to and from the wedding locale is not necessary (and an additional expense), but guests would surely appreciate the hospitality of shuttle buses or luxury coaches to take them to the wedding festivities, especially if the wedding location is a little off the beaten path. Shuttles are also great because it is like a big car pool, cutting down on vehicles on the road and therefore carbon emissions.

You should designate times and meeting locations at the guests' hotels and provide a timeline for arrivals and departures. Arrangements like this make sure your guests get to the ceremony and reception on time, and as an added bonus, no one will have to worry about driving after partaking in some wine and champagne.

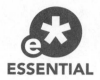
Prepare a travel package with all the phone numbers, websites, and other vital information that the guests will need to plan their trip. Shortly after getting engaged, make the necessary arrangements with the airlines and hotels and send this information to your guests with the Save the Date, or as a separate mailing.

Hotels

As with airfare or other travel arrangements, the couple is not expected to pay for hotel accommodations. You should, however, arrange for discounted or group lodging for your out-of-town attendants. It is a great idea to contact the sales offices of local hotels in varying price ranges. Arrange to reserve a block of rooms for your guests, and you can lock in a discounted rate for a particular period of time. Just be sure the guests know when your special rate expires.

Hotel room blocks can provide your guests a great deal, but great deals can be found online. Of course, there is no guarantee of that. A hotel room block will generally reserve a set number of rooms for a set price up until thirty days prior to the wedding.

Check the local area to see if there are any hotels or other accommodations in the general area that are vegan friendly or eco-friendly. Many areas have at least one boutique-style hotel that fits the bill. You may not be able to find a purely vegan hotel, but finding one that offers vegan meal options, is not furnished with leather sofas, and is environmentally conscious is a good choice.

A Good Group

There is a lot to be said for selecting a "host" hotel. When the guests are gathered at a specific hotel, they can enjoy the following:

- The guest can mingle with other guests during downtime.
- You can help create a carpool option for those guests who are staying at one locale. It promotes friendship and is eco-friendly.
- It is easier to arrange for group transportation if the guests are located at one or maybe two locales.

Keep in mind that some guests may not be able to afford or feel comfortable in the hotel you select and may choose to find their own accommodations. Try to provide one or two hotels with different price points in the same general area. Other guests may have preferred hotels due to mileage or travel points, and some may just want their privacy. Do your best to provide the information, but ultimately the decision is up to the guest.

A Warm Welcome

Guests who attend your wedding are making an effort to be there to witness this cherished moment in your life. After traveling, there could be nothing more wonderful than arriving at your destination and being welcomed with open arms. It is a wonderful, welcoming gesture to provide the guests with a list of activities and some genuine hospitality to make this a wedding and a trip they will never forget.

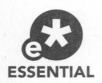

ESSENTIAL

Put together a list of vegan-friendly restaurants and attractions in the area. Vegans will love this and nonvegans can acquaint themselves with the vegan way of life in the area if they choose.

Hospitality

Imagine the guests' delight when they enter their hotel room and find a hospitality package of travel amenities and/or snacks from the bride and groom. These are not necessary, but the guests appreciate them, and they make a great impression. And it is a great way to introduce them to some yummy vegan snacks and products.

What's in Them

The hospitality packages can be as simple as bottled water and snacks or they can be more elaborate, including gourmet food selections and wine. Your packages can be created to reflect your wedding destination or theme as well, for example, a bottle of wine for a wine-country wedding or beach towels and flip flops for a beachfront destination. A wedding activities guide or itinerary and a local travel guide are also great additions. Other items you may want to include are: cookies, gum or mints, nuts, crackers, vegan chocolates, trail mix, and dried or fresh fruit.

You will need one package per room, but be sure to include the appropriate number of items, such as water bottles, to accommodate the number of guests in the room. Call the hotels to confirm the number of booked rooms so that you can prepare the packages. You can create the packages yourself or order them from a basket or gift company.

Get Me to the Church on Time

Picture this: It's your wedding day. You're all dressed and ready to go, and all you need now is the limousine to roll up and get you to the church on time. But it doesn't. Or it does come, but it's covered by a dusty haze and has mud caked on its three remaining hubcaps. Or it looks snazzy enough on the outside, but inside, the television and bar you requested are not to be found. You wouldn't mind any of that, would you?

Advanced Reservations

Generally speaking, it's never too early to look into your transportation options. If you're getting married during the peak season (April–October), get on the ball right away. It's not uncommon for limos to be booked a year in advance; many companies will even take reservations up to a year and a half before an event. If you're unsure about your area (limos don't seem to be very popular, or there just aren't a lot of weddings), call some companies and ask for their recommendations.

Keep in mind that May and June are also big prom and graduation months, and that limos will be in high demand for these events. As soon as you start thinking about your wedding day transportation, get moving on booking your vehicles.

ALERT

It is common for luxury cars to have leather interior and trim. What's a good vegan to do? Ask the company about the interiors of their cars, and ask if they have alternative cars without leather seating. If they don't, look elsewhere or decide how important this is to you.

Deal with the Owner

Try to find a company that owns its limousines. Owners are more likely to keep track of a car's maintenance and whereabouts. You do not want to ride in a limo that has seen its share of unauthorized excursions. Additionally, you want to also:

- Make sure you verify a service's license and insurance coverage.
- Get references.
- Inspect all of the cars. Does the fleet look modern and up to date, or are the cars creaking and groaning and looking like they just might be on their last legs? Are there obvious scratches or dents on the cars? (There shouldn't be.)

- When you get in to inspect the vehicles, are the interior surfaces spotless? (They should be.) Are the windows clean? Do the cars smell like smoke? Is there enough room for your groom and his linebacker buddies to spread out without crushing any crinolines? Is there enough headroom for the gigantic hairdos your bridesmaids will be sporting?
- Most importantly, does this company have the kind of limo you want? If you only want a certain color car, are they willing to guarantee that? Don't take a company's word that it can get you a black stretch limo without black leather interior. You need to see it with your own eyes—and don't sign anything until you have.
- Is the limousine outfitted in leather interior and trim? Are there options either with this company or elsewhere?

Some limo services rent cars out from another company, which means those cars are probably being shared by several other services, too. In addition to maintenance and overuse problems, it's harder for a company that doesn't own its own limos to ensure the availability of any given car, or to supply you with a car of the color and size you want.

Questions to Ask

To ensure that you'll be getting quality transportation for your money, you should ask certain questions of any company you rent transportation from. (Note: The following list of questions is geared toward limousine rental, but it will give you an idea of the kind of information you should get from any transportation supplier.)

○ What are the rates? (Most limousine services charge by the hour. Unfortunately for you, the clock starts ticking the minute they leave their home base rather than when you start using the vehicle.)
○ What is the company's cancellation policy?
○ Is there a required minimum fee or number of rental hours?
○ When does the clock start on the rental?

○ What is the policy on tipping? Is it included in the hourly rate, or should we account for it separately? (You won't want to tip your chauffeur at the end of the night if the gratuity is covered in the fee you paid. It's doubtful the service will be so spectacular that you'll want to pay twice!)

○ How much of a deposit is required to reserve the vehicle(s) for our wedding? When is the final payment due?

○ Will the company provide champagne? Ice? Glasses? A television? Will these items cost extra?

How Much?

Most limousine services charge by the hour. Many companies have package deals with a specific number of hours included in the price, but you need to understand what's included. A three-hour deal might sound like more than enough time, since you know you're not going to be sitting in that limo for three hours. But if there's a delay between the ceremony and the reception—if you're getting married at one o'clock and your reception is at five, for example—you're going to need at least four-and-a-half hours.

Sign Here

Once you decide on a limousine service, get all the details finalized in a written contract. It should specify the type of car, additional options and services you will need, the expected length of service, the date, and the time. If there's a specific limo you just have to have, ask the owner to specify it on the contract. Some limo companies have vanity plates on their cars for this very purpose. If the car you want has a plate that reads Limo A-1, there will be very little chance of Limo B-1 showing up at your house on your wedding day, as long as everything's in writing.

Ask about contingencies. If you're choosing the company's top-of-the-line car and something happens to it, what then? Get this in writing, also.

ALERT

It's a good idea to arrange for the limo to arrive at least fifteen to thirty minutes before you're going to need it, just to be on the safe side. This way, if the driver gets caught in traffic, you won't be forced to hitchhike to the ceremony.

Limousine Optional

Think about the entrance you want to make at your wedding ceremony. How do you picture it? Are you dropping from the sky in a hot-air balloon? Rolling by on a parade float? Or panting up to the door in your most comfortable sneakers after an invigorating run? These days, very little is off limits as far as wedding transportation goes. Innovative couples have been known to use helicopters, boats, hot rods, antique cars, Lear jets, motorcycles . . . as long as it can move you from here to there, it's okay for your wedding.

Some of the most popular—and easy-to-find—alternatives are:

- **Town cars.** A town car is a smaller chauffeur-driven option. Generally, town cars can be rented for shorter periods of time. They generally accommodate only two passengers, but may just be the perfect way to get you and the groom to and from the festivities, at a lesser cost.
- **Shuttles and trolleys.** Shuttles and trolleys may not provide you with that sleek wow factor, but they are functional and, nowadays, nicely equipped. There are plenty of seats for everyone; plenty of room for purses, coats, and champagne bottles; and a fun, casual atmosphere on board. Trolleys or even double-decker buses offer a unique transportation experience. Many trolley rides are open-air affairs, but in colder climates, most offer some kind of protection from the winter elements.

FACT

Another option for a summer or warm-climate wedding is renting a convertible for you and your groom to escape in. Is there a better picture of a fun-filled wedding than this? Of course, if you're paying an outrageous amount to have your hair done that morning, this may not be your best option.

Free Ride

If for some reason you are unable to rent wedding transportation, look around for family and friends who have nice big cars they'd be willing to lend you. (Years ago, this was actually how brides and grooms got around on their wedding days—imagine!) Some car buffs are likely to be horrified at the idea of someone else behind the wheel of their baby. If that's the case, you can always ask them to play the part of chauffeur for the day. The only requirement here is that the cars have to be clean. You should pay for the prewedding car wash and detailing. And be sure to remember your generous friends with a little gift and a full tank of gas.

Can We Hitch a Ride?

You are also responsible for providing or arranging transportation for the members of your wedding party. You might also want to make sure your parents and the groom's parents won't be standing on the corner waiting for a bus to the ceremony. If your budget allows, consider renting an extra limousine or two to chauffeur them to and from the ceremony and reception sites. Otherwise, arrange for those with the nicest cars to transport the rest of the group. Make sure everyone is aware of who's taking whom, what time people will have to be ready, and where they may have to meet.

Environmentally Friendly Transportation

Motor vehicles account for a huge portion of the carbon dioxide emissions that contribute to global warming, and they also release other toxic pollutants into the atmosphere. Growing awareness of this is forcing vehicle manufacturers to become greener, and people are making more environmentally friendly choices when it comes to their transportation, not just for their weddings, but for everyday living.

The high cost of gasoline and increasing awareness of the political ramifications of dependence on foreign oil makes gas-guzzling SUVs less attractive, and more and more drivers are turning in their SUVs for more fuel-efficient cars. Be creative, and you can have fun and functionally green transportation without giving up on style.

Arrive in Eco-Style

You can have uniquely green transportation for every aspect of your wedding—for the commute between ceremony and reception locations (if there is one) or for your departure as the newly married couple. Eco-friendly vehicles such as hybrids and electric cars are practical for getting from one place to another. You can also consider vehicles that run on alternative fuels such as biodiesel and E85.

Hybrids run on a gasoline engine and an electric motor. The electric motor is powered by a battery that recharges itself by capturing the energy that is released whenever the brakes are applied. According to hybridcars.com, United States oil consumption could be reduced by 1.5 million barrels a day if fuel efficiency were increased by just five miles per gallon.

Green for Everyone

For all your guests and everyone in your wedding party, you could arrange for carpooling or shuttling from one location to another. Many rental companies are now offering greener choices by adding hybrids in their rental fleet. Consider shuttle buses that run on biodiesel, or offer guests information on renting hybrid vehicles. If the ceremony and reception sites are close together, just walk from one venue to the next. To keep things even greener, have the ceremony and reception in the same locale.

Even limousine rental companies are expanding their green efforts and offering a greener variety of luxury. Every day, more companies are realizing that they have to be more environmentally friendly and offer responsible options for their customers. Custom-built hybrid limos are available through some companies, and in the near future the ultimate in luxurious rides may come in a green model. Bentley has announced plans to develop an eco-friendly limo. With a little bit of effort, a few phone calls, and maybe some web surfing, you should be able to find a green vehicle so you can ride around on your wedding day in eco-style.

CHAPTER 18

The Wedding Puzzle

That magical day that seemed as though it was so far away is right around the corner. By this point, your plans are in place, but they may look like one giant wedding-planning puzzle. The pieces are all there, but how do they fit together? Now is the time to regroup, reorganize, seat your guests, and pull together an itinerary. When you do this, you will see how the pieces fit together, and how your vision comes to life.

Have a Seat

Trying to come up with a seating plan that pleases everyone seems like an impossible task, but rest assured it does all work out . . . eventually. A seating plan takes some work, and unfortunately, it is one of the last tasks to complete, as you must wait until all the responses are in before you can finalize it. Realize that no matter how hard you try, someone—your mother, your fiancé's mother, your cousin, even your fiancé—is bound to have an opinion. You may feel like giving up, but don't despair; it really does all work out.

ALERT

Single guests may already feel like they have a sign pointing out, "Hey, look, I'm single!" When doing the seating plan, mix the single guests in with the couples, seating three to four singles at each table, and try not to seat a lone single guest at a table of couples. Finally, remember, your wedding is not the time to play matchmaker.

Like-Minded Seating

Before you set the seating chart into motion, you may need to take your wedding menu into account as you seat the guests at the reception. If you have chosen to serve a vegetarian option or even an organic animal protein in addition to the vegan fare, sitting the vegans together, the vegetarians together, and the meat eaters together may be helpful.

ESSENTIAL

Of course, there is always the chance that a vegan is married to a meat eater. In that case, you know your guests best and seating them together is called for. The vegan is probably used to sharing meals with her meat-eating spouse, so this will not offend her.

The caterer won't care so much about who sits where, but surely any strictly vegan friends would find it more comfortable to be sitting at a table with others who are not consuming any animal product. If one has such strong beliefs, sharing a table with those eating animal protein may just turn their stomachs. Of course, the smell of the beef or chicken may be in the room, but that is entirely different than staring at it for the duration of the meal. The vegetarians may feel the same way. Chances are the meat eaters won't even notice.

How to Do It

A seating plan falls just short of being considered a necessity, but it is a courtesy and convenience for your guests. Guests, especially those who don't know many people, often feel uncomfortable without assigned seating. If you're planning a cocktail party or not planning to serve a full meal, a seating plan isn't necessary, but you should have enough tables and chairs to accommodate all of your guests.

These simple steps will help you as you continue to pull together the seating chart.

SIMPLE STEPS FOR SEATING

- Get a floor plan from the venue. It should outline the layout of the room (dance floor, bar, guest book, gift table, etc.).
- You need to decide where you will be sitting as well as where the other tables of honor with the wedding party and your families will be positioned.
- Ask how many guests may be seated at each table. A general rule is eight to ten guests at a 60" round table. This will determine the number of tables you will need for dining.
- Decide if you are going to solicit input from your families when determining who should sit where.
- Begin matching guests up by families, where you know them from, or by similar interests. From here you will be playing a card game of sorts, mixing and matching until you have the right guests at the right seats.
- Optional, if you are providing other, nonvegan meal options: Seat vegans with vegans, etc.

Place Cards and Escort Cards

The easiest way to indicate the guests' table assignments is to have escort cards situated near the reception room entrance. Guests would pick up the escort card to find their table assignment. If you are only assigning guests to a table, they may then find any seat they wish at that table. If you would like to designate a place setting, you will also need to place cards on the table.

FACT

The term "place card" is often misused when referring to an escort card. An escort card is a small card that a guest will pick up as she enters the reception. It directs the guest to her table. A place card would be placed on the dining table, designating the place where the guest should sit.

If you're planning a very formal wedding, both escort cards and place cards are called for. At less formal receptions, escort cards can be used to indicate the guests' assigned tables, but you should use place cards at the head table.

Green Place Cards

If you decide to use place cards, let them be multipurpose. Let the place card and favor be one and the same. Some ideas for place cards that can be favors as well include:

- Seed packets with the guests' names written elegantly on the package
- A small potted plant with a guest's name on the pot
- Plantable place cards made with handcrafted seed paper
- A piece of fruit with a little card attached made from handmade, recycled, or tree-free paper
- A bar of handmade soap with the guest's name carved into it
- A handmade paper envelope containing bath salts
- A small package of handmade note cards tied with hemp, organic cotton ribbon, or twine

- A card made from handmade, recycled, or tree-free paper, announcing that charitable donations have been made to the bride and groom's charity of choice in place of favors
- Bags or envelopes made from sustainable materials filled with fresh or dried organic herbs
- Photo frames made of green materials

Places of Honor

The head table is wherever the bride and groom sit, and is, understandably, the focus of the reception. It usually faces the other tables, is front and center in the room, and near the dance floor. The table is situated to allow guests a perfect view of you and your groom. While the tradition of a head table is still followed, there are now many other options for the bride and groom when it comes to seating.

The Head Table

Traditionally, the bride and groom, honor attendants, bridesmaids, and groomsmen sit at the head table. The bride and groom sit in the middle, with the groom on the bride's left, the best man next to the bride, and the maid of honor next to the groom. The ushers and bridesmaids then sit on alternating sides of the bride and groom. Child attendants should sit at a regular table with their parents.

Reserved for the Bride and Groom

A very popular alternative for bride and groom seating is the sweetheart table, which is a table just for two . . . you and your new husband. Many couples prefer this option, as it lets them have a little time together to eat their meal, and it also allows the attendants to sit with their spouses or significant others.

ESSENTIAL

As the bride and groom, you are stars of the show, but you need to eat, too. Arrange in advance for your venue or caterer to serve your meal, salad, and main course first, so that you may eat and be ready to greet your guests and participate in other activities.

The Wedding Party

If there is no head table, most of the time the wedding party would sit at one or two guest tables designated for them. They could also sit with their spouses throughout the room. Sometimes, although not done as often, a long table is set up behind the sweetheart table and the wedding party will sit there, kind of like a head table without the bride and groom.

The Family

The head table is usually reserved for the members of the wedding party; parents usually sit at separate tables with their families. There's no single correct seating arrangement for the parents, however. The bride's and groom's parents can sit together with the officiant and his spouse at the parents' table, or each set of parents can host their own table with family and friends. If your parents decide to include separate parents' tables, be sure that one of them includes the officiant and his spouse.

Don't Sit There!

By this point, you have probably already realized that planning a wedding requires a little extra maneuvering if you have divorced parents. If you're lucky, either your parents get along or have agreed to declare a truce for a day. If you're not so lucky, seating arrangements can be a bit tricky. But as always, these problems can be solved through communication and flexibility.

Divorced Parents

You shouldn't seat your divorced parents at the same table, no matter how well they get along; people may get the wrong idea about their marital status. If you're having a parents' table, have the parent who raised you sit with your in-laws and the officiant, and seat your other parent with his or her own family and friends. Or, you can seat each parent at his or her own table with family and friends.

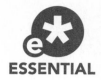

ESSENTIAL

If divorce has caused friction in the family, you should seat the said parties as far away from each other as possible in order to minimize interaction. Try to place both tables in equally desirable positions near the head table, but on opposite sides of the room.

The Attendants' Spouses

It is an age-old question—where do the attendants' spouses sit? Well, they can sit at tables with the other guests, preferably near the head table area. Spouses don't usually sit at the head table with their husbands or wives. If you are choosing to have a sweetheart table, you can seat the spouses together.

Rowdy Guests

Rowdy guest may become the life of the party as the night wears on, but they are not necessarily the group you want front and center. Put their table/tables on the opposite side of the room from the bar, and don't place them front and center, so that they won't be a spectacle if they drink too much. Also, tell the bartender that no shots are to be served at your wedding, or have a soft bar only.

Seating the Kids

You've made the decision that kids are a go at your wedding. Now you need to figure out where to seat them. Not only do you need a seating plan that allows comfort and flexibility for both the kids and their parents, you really need to figure out how to keep them happy during the reception.

If there will be a number of children at the reception, a kid's table is a great way for both the kids and the parents to enjoy themselves. If there are only a couple of children, you may just want to keep them with their parents. Children age seven-plus are typically old enough to eat dinner at a table with the other kids. Of course, think about the placement of the kids' tables and where the parents' tables are. Consider grouping those guests with kids in one area of the venue and placing the kids' tables in that same area. You can also mix the kids up by ages, so that some older children will be available to assist the younger children.

FACT

If there will be small children attending, be sure to ask the venue if they have high chairs or booster chairs on hand. If they don't, rent some. It will be a small cost but a huge convenience for your guests. You may want to consider purchasing some cute bibs and kid utensils as well—parents can forget these items, and venues rarely have them on hand.

Seating the Vendors

Your wedding vendors need to eat, too! The caterer generally offers a lesser priced meal to accommodate these needs, but where are they supposed to sit? Having vendors sit in empty seats with the guests is the least desirable option for both the vendors and the guests. It can make the guests feel like they were seated at a B-list table, and the vendor really could use a break from the action. If the vendor table cannot be set up outside of the dining room, a vendor table in the back of the room is perfectly fine. In this situation, all of the vendors know where to find their meal and are out of the way of the guests.

ALERT

Be sure to allot at least thirty minutes in the timeline for the vendors to eat and take a break. Provide them with their meal and nonalcoholic beverages. Professional vendors know what it takes to perform well at their jobs, and they will not disappoint you. Many work with assistants, so that while one eats, the other can cover the activities.

Where to Go, What to Do

Where to go, how to get there, and when to be there—essential information that the wedding party, your parents, and the vendors all need to know. As the wedding day approaches, not only do you have paperwork to fill out and timelines to plan, but most importantly, you need to communicate this to all of the involved parties. A well-planned itinerary is the perfect way to do this.

The Itinerary

The day draws nearer. Are you wondering about the who, what, where of the day? Well, the itinerary is here to keep everyone abreast of the important places and events for the people involved in the wedding. It is essentially a schedule for the wedding day that includes detailed entries organized by time. Usually, the itinerary begins with the bride's first event of the day, getting her hair and makeup styled, and ends with the couple leaving the reception. The itinerary should list each person by name in accordance with the times they are to arrive and where they are to be.

Creating an Itinerary

If you have been working with a wedding planner, she is most likely going to do this for you, with your input, of course. Discuss this with her and make sure this is one of the responsibilities you hired her to assist with. If you do not have a wedding planner, you will be in charge of the itinerary. You will work with the vendor contracts you have that state arrival and departure times, and with your ceremony and reception venues, for which you already have set times booked. These key pieces of information are the starting point for creating an itinerary.

FACT

Begin the outline for your itinerary about four to six weeks prior to the wedding. This allows enough time to create a schedule and make changes as you verify details and timing. Once the itinerary is complete, make copies and pass them out to the wedding party, families, readers, soloists, and any other people helping at the wedding.

Here are a few simple steps to get you started on your itinerary:

- Start with the established start times of the ceremony and reception. Use these times to work forward and backward, filling in the additional confirmed times in the schedule.

- Confirm arrival and setup times with the ceremony and/or reception venues.
- Know how long it takes to travel between all locations. Account for travel time, and schedule departure and arrival times.
- Schedule the times for preceremony events such as hair and makeup and photo sessions.
- Confirm arrival and departure times with the vendors. Be sure the order and timing makes sense. For example, if you are scheduling photographs to begin at the hotel, before going to the church, make sure the florist delivers the bouquets to the hotel and not the church.
- Decide on what traditions you want to incorporate into the ceremony and reception, and include specific details such as song titles, names of those proposing toasts, who will be dancing, etc.
- Review the reception itinerary with the location manager and then the entertainment. Confirm that the timing for the formalities (grand entrance, toast, first dance, etc.) will work within the timeframe for the meal service.
- Create a schedule with the photographer. Heed his advice when preparing this schedule; he's done this before and knows how long it takes.
- Include wedding day contact names, office phone numbers, and cell phone numbers for all vendors.
- Include detailed information on décor and setup plans: linen colors, table favor placement, where escort cards are to be set up, etc.

ALERT

No matter how much you plan and prepare, you must remember the itinerary represents the best-case scenario. This is what you want to have happen and when you want it to happen, but on your wedding day, you may have to depart from the itinerary to accommodate delays and changes. Don't fret. Be flexible! It will all work out.

Calling to Confirm

After planning so carefully and spending so much money to create the perfect wedding day, now is not the time to let any details slip through the cracks. As the day draws nearer, calling and e-mailing each vendor to finalize details, including the wedding day itinerary, will provide you with peace of mind and the assurance your wedding is right on track.

Paperwork

Go through your signed contracts and paperwork and make a calendar showing when each vendor needs their payments and any necessary paperwork. Among other things, the DJ or band needs your list of musical selections, the caterer needs a guest count, and the baker needs to know exactly how many guests are coming as well as what flavors you have finally decided upon.

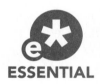

ESSENTIAL

Most vendors require final payments about two weeks prior to the wedding day. A select few may let you pay them on the wedding day. Check your contracts to verify payment dates and how each vendor requests payment. Some vendors will not accept credit cards for final payments; some will only accept a money order or cash if paid on the wedding day.

Follow-Up

As you finalize details and such, there is much to be said for actually speaking with the vendor. E-mail, texts, and voicemails have their place, but cannot replace good old-fashioned communication. As the big day gets closer, you should supply each vendor with a copy of the itinerary, so that they know what to expect. Follow up your phone conversation with a quick e-mail (or fax) that includes a brief update on anything you spoke about and a copy of the itinerary. Of course, if you make any changes to your services or products, there should be written confirmation as well.

Wedding Day Prep

You've planned, you've confirmed, you've planned some more. All that's left to do is get married, or so it seems. There are some final preparations for the wedding day that still need to be tended to. So, get going; there are things to pack, copies to make, and places to go.

A Place for Everything

Every bride tends to accumulate a lot of wedding stuff—programs, place cards, and favors, to mention just a few. The last thing you want to do on your wedding day is be responsible for hauling bags and boxes of wedding paraphernalia to the church and reception. The first thing you need to do is sort the items; putting the ceremony items together and the reception items together.

Ask your wedding planner if you can bring these items to her a day or two prior to the wedding or at the rehearsal and have her deliver/be responsible for getting the items to the correct venue. If there is no wedding planner, ask the location managers for the ceremony and reception if they have a secure room or area where these items can be stored. If neither of these options work, ask a very trustworthy friend to assist you with delivering these items on the wedding day.

ESSENTIAL

Amenity baskets are a great treat for the guests. Make small baskets with aspirins, hairspray, mouthwash, mints, shoeshine towels, bobby pins, and other necessities and place the baskets in the restroom at the reception. It really looks like you are trying to take care of the guests' every need, just as a good host should.

Wedding Day Accessories

Following is a checklist of wedding day accessories. Keep in mind, that this is a generic checklist. Your particular wedding may have more or less accessories as well as other specialty items; just add them in, check them off, and you are ready for the wedding day.

WEDDING ACCESSORY CHECKLIST

○ Aisle runner
○ Bubbles, rose petals, etc. (for tossing or sendoff)
○ Cake knife and server
○ Cake topper
○ Cash and envelopes (for last-minute tips and expenses)
○ Card box (for gift table)
○ Centerpieces
○ Copies of itinerary, vendors' contracts, vendor contact numbers, seating chart
○ Decorations
○ Engagement photos
○ Favors
○ Flower girl basket
○ Guest book
○ Pens for guest book
○ Place cards
○ Ring pillow
○ Table numbers
○ Toasting flutes
○ Unity candle
○ Wedding programs

ALERT

Guests are always misplacing their escort cards. Bring at least two copies of the seating list to have on hand at the reception. The lists should be typed out in alphabetical order and each person's table assignment should also be included.

It's a Bridal Emergency!

When you are moments away from walking down the aisle and you need a safety pin to keep a hem up or a mint to get rid of dragon breath, your problems are easily solved and a bridal emergency is avoided with a well-stocked emergency kit. This is one wedding accessory that no bride should be without. A carefully packed kit that includes simple everyday items as well as wedding-specific items is a lifesaver for you and the guests.

The Kit

Telling the wedding party to come prepared is great, but this is your wedding, and as such, it is best you take action. An emergency kit is not only for the wedding party; it is really for everyone at the wedding. You never know when a guest might need some antacid or some aspirin. The kit can also be made to accommodate your wedding colors (by adding thread to match the bridesmaids' gowns) and even the location. For example, if you are marrying on a ranch without a lot of night lighting, flashlights would be an important addition.

ESSENTIAL

After you have packed the main emergency kit, prepare a smaller one just for the groom and his men. He can have it with him in case he has his own emergency, and won't have to worry about getting a glimpse of (or worrying) you.

The Bridal Emergency Kit Checklist

Oftentimes, a mother or bridesmaid goes about packing this kit as a special surprise. However, you, the vegan bride, may want to take control of this kit yourself to ensure all the products are cruelty free and vegan friendly. You may have some specific items here and there, but below are some basic contents of a bridal emergency kit.

BRIDAL EMERGENCY KIT
- ❍ Aspirin or ibuprofen
- ❍ Baby or talcum powder
- ❍ Bobby pins
- ❍ Bottled water
- ❍ Breath mints
- ❍ Cellophane tape

- ⭘ Clean white cloth (for dabbing off stains on wedding dress)
- ⭘ Clear bandages or liquid bandage
- ⭘ Clear nail polish
- ⭘ Corsage pins
- ⭘ Crackers, energy bars, etc. (all vegan)
- ⭘ Deodorant
- ⭘ Double-stick tape
- ⭘ Duct tape (one regular and one in white)
- ⭘ Extra stockings
- ⭘ Facial tissue or handkerchief
- ⭘ Glue (super glue, hot glue, and hot glue gun—vegan brands)
- ⭘ Hairspray
- ⭘ Money
- ⭘ Mouthwash
- ⭘ Nail glue
- ⭘ Nail polish (to match your shade for a quick touch-up)
- ⭘ Rubber bands
- ⭘ Sanitary napkins/tampons
- ⭘ Scissors
- ⭘ Sewing kit (including straight pins, needle, and thread. Bring white and black thread. Don't forget a color to match the bridesmaids' dresses and the groomsmen's accessories.)
- ⭘ Spot remover
- ⭘ Static-cling spray
- ⭘ Toothbrush and toothpaste
- ⭘ Tweezers
- ⭘ White chalk (for concealing dirt smudges)

CHAPTER 19

Trip of a Lifetime

With all the frenzied coordinating, organizing, and worrying
involved, getting yourself married can be a full-time job—
and then some! When it's all over, you'll need more than
just an ordinary vacation to recuperate. On the surface,
a honeymoon is no different from any other vacation you
might take, but to a pair of newlyweds, the honeymoon is
a much-anticipated getaway. This once-in-a-lifetime trip is
the grand finale of your wedding, and the reward for your
careful planning . . . and a chance to support socially conscious travel.

Decisions! Decisions!

Like the wedding venues and vendors, some of the most sought-after destinations may be booked up to a year in advance, so begin your planning early. When you do research honeymoon destinations, don't get locked into what you think a honeymoon has to be. A honeymoon can be anything you want, from backpacking across Europe to lounging on a beach in the Caribbean to camping in the mountains.

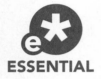

ESSENTIAL

Check local vegan associations, blogs, and message boards for areas that offer vegan fare and/or cater to vegans. It will be much easier for you to enjoy your honeymoon if not all of your time is spent searching out vegan meals and supplies once you arrive.

As you plan, remember almost any destination can accommodate your vegan lifestyle. It merely takes some forethought and planning to accomplish this.

Here is a list of the easiest and simplest to-dos to get your honeymoon off on the cruelty-free foot:

- Do a quick search on the web. Use key words like "vegan restaurant (insert location)" or "vegan hotel (insert location)." This will easily pull up vegan restaurants and locales in the area you are considering.
- Be sure to pack everything vegan that you need. Don't count on local shops having vegan toothpaste, lotions, birth control, etc. Use the packing list later in this chapter to double check yourself.
- Call and or e-mail the hotel/resort as well as the chef and explain your needs. Ask what they can do to facilitate a vegan experience at their establishment.

FACT

VegNews is a print and online resource for all things vegan. Visit their website and search "travel" or "honeymoons" to explore a world of options for your vegan honeymoon.

Where Are We Going?

You might have your honeymoon all planned out in your head right now (you know, the one you've been imagining since you were ten years old). However, your groom might have vastly different ideas. First, you'll need to pinpoint what each of you expects from this trip. Does he want to golf or fish or ski? Are you looking to see some shows, do some shopping, or sit by the pool? Each of you is allowed to insist on the inclusion of one activity (other than snuggling up to each other, that is). And if this doesn't help, you'll either have to plan a two-part honeymoon, or, more realistically, you'll have to find a happy compromise.

ALERT

Honeymoon or not, everyone has their limits. You don't want your honeymoon to be marred by an argument over who's calling all the shots. Make sure whatever you're planning is going to keep both of you entertained for the entire vacation.

Fair and Square

Keep in mind that the activities you're planning should be enjoyable to both of you. Many couples plan their honeymoon by saying to one another, "Whatever you want is fine with me," until one partner takes that ball and runs with it. The ensuing honeymoon turns out to be filled with activities that the planner finds interesting. And even though he or she may have genuinely thought that his or her spouse would enjoy the various outings, the nonplanner ends up bored or annoyed instead.

It's fair to expect a certain amount of compromise on your honeymoon. For example, you might want to introduce your groom to waterskiing, a sport you mastered long ago. But you can't expect your spouse to spend the entire week giving in to your every demand. After all, this is his honeymoon, too. Likewise, if you really despise museums and your new husband loves to spend the day looking at abstract art, you might agree to accompany him for a day or two, but after that, chances are you'd be bored and a little miffed.

Money Talks

Ultimately, of course, your budget is likely to have at least as big an influence on your choice of destination as your dreams. Consult a travel agent or the Internet to find low-priced airfares, reduced-rate package deals, and other ways to save money. You may be pleasantly surprised. Perhaps you can afford a trip to Hawaii by staying at a less than four-star hotel, or travel Europe via hostels and bed and breakfasts. Remember, however, to confirm that inexpensive lodging does not mean without running water, dilapidated, or situated in the red-light district (though all of these situations, in their own way, may add some excitement to your trip).

Some couples choose to postpone the trip for several months, either for financial reasons or because one partner just can't get the vacation time from work right after the wedding. If you're still in the early stages of planning your wedding and you just know that you won't be able to afford any sort of honeymoon, your travel agent might be able to help you by setting up a honeymoon registry.

You and your groom need to decide what you'd like to do or see on your honeymoon and narrow down your choices from there. Obviously, some areas have more to offer than others. If you think you'd like to see a particular region on your honeymoon, but you aren't 100 percent sure about it, do some research on the region. This is something you should do anyway, no matter where you choose to go. Ask your travel agent for some brochures, or look online for the city's chamber of commerce website.

Sealing the Deal

Perhaps you're used to handling your vacation arrangements by yourself, without anyone's help. Or maybe you have a great travel agent and you'd never make a move without her. No matter which method you prefer, make sure you start early enough to book the hotels, activities, and flights that you want. If you are planning on having a green or eco-honeymoon, be sure to check into any particulars on timing or schedules as soon as possible.

Book It!

If you're making your own travel arrangements and you're taking off soon after your wedding, don't forget that your plane tickets should be booked in your maiden name. You'll need a valid photo ID to board your flight, and the name on the ID must match the name on your ticket.

Also, if you're taking off immediately following the reception (or the morning after), try to arrange for smooth travel connections. As you're looking at tickets online, an eight-hour layover may seem like a bit of a hassle, but you may think you're willing to accept it for the sake of saving a few hundred bucks. But keep in mind that you're likely to be exhausted and anxious to get on with the honeymoonin'—and a long layover (or a series of them) on the day after your wedding might get your trip off on the wrong foot. Fatigue can breed irritability and forgetfulness. Add the stress of travel to that, and you have the recipe for potential disaster. Even if you get to your destination without mishap, you certainly don't want to risk bickering with your spouse your first full day as a married couple. Moods could swing, tears may be shed, and you'll lose almost an entire day to travel in the process.

ALERT

If either of you is generally not a good traveler, you might want to keep things as close to home as possible. You could find a nice resort that's within driving distance, for example, instead of hopping flight after flight, which will only add to any travel-related misery.

If possible, try to get at least six hours of sleep the night before you take off. You may not wake up totally refreshed (given that weddings have a way of making you feel like you've run a marathon), but you'll be better off than if you only slept for two hours. Make some time for a long, hot shower and a hearty breakfast, and you should have a good start to the first day of your honeymoon.

Using Travel Agents

Maybe you scoff at the very idea of travel agents, reasoning that you can do all of this yourself. If you're going out of the country, however, you might benefit from working with an agent who can enlighten you as to the finer points of international travel. Because foreign vacations can get very complicated—with connecting flights that have to meet boats that have to meet trains—putting all the responsibility into the hands of a trained professional might be a good idea. After all, you've already got enough to think about with planning the wedding.

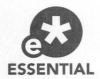

ESSENTIAL

Depending on where you go and if your airline offers a meal, be sure to request a vegan meal option for the trip, and be sure to plan plenty of your own vegan snacks for the ride.

Your agent will be able to tell you which paperwork, identification, and other necessities you will need in order to travel abroad; basically, expect that if you are leaving the country, you need a passport. (More on passports later in this chapter.) Documents you will need to track down if you're planning on leaving the country include:

- Birth certificate
- Driver's license (or other picture ID)
- Proof of marriage
- Proof of citizenship

Travel agents are also on the ball as far as alerting you to potential troubles. You might not want to risk traveling to a spot during its rainy season. Or you might find out from your agent, who's in the know, that your four-star resort is planning on adding another entire wing during your stay, which will add up to lots of round-the-clock noise. This would be enough to make you want to stay across town. Nowadays, some foreign countries post travel alerts for Americans, which you'll obviously want to know about before you attempt to board a plane to a restricted or dangerous area.

Of course, you can find this information on your own, but it will take a considerable amount of time to research the things that your travel agent already knows. Just consider whether the time it will take is worth it, or if it could be better spent focusing on the wedding itself.

Passports

Passports are relatively easy to obtain—as long as you're not an international spy. You'll need to give yourself a minimum of six weeks, but you should really start the process as soon as you can to avoid any last-minute problems. It is possible to pay extra (somewhere in the range of an arm and a leg) for expedited service, which generally takes about two weeks.

Your first step is to fill out an application, which can be found online at *www.state.gov/travel*. If you're applying for the first time, you'll have to take the application to a passport agency or a passport acceptance facility. This isn't as hard as it sounds—many of these facilities are located inside of larger post offices, some libraries, and county offices. You'll bring proof of U.S. citizenship (your birth certificate or naturalization certificate will do); a photo ID (such as a valid driver's license or government ID); two passport photos (which can be taken at many one-hour photo shops); your Social Security number; and money (the fee currently totals $85).

Do Your Homework

Before you take off on any vacation, you should acquaint yourself with the area you're traveling to. If you're going to Chicago, for example, you won't need to rent a car, because public transportation is around every corner, and you'll never find a parking spot, anyway. If you're headed to New York City, you'd better start studying the subway system, unless you want to drop a fortune in cab fare. If you're going to land in a foreign airport, get yourself a map of its layout so that you'll know where to find the baggage claim and where you'll have to go to grab a taxi.

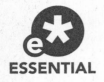

Know what kind of weather to expect. You're headed to the Caribbean, you say, and all you're going to need is a bikini and some sunscreen (you freckle so badly!). But if you're vacationing during hurricane season, you might want to bring a raincoat . . . and inquire as to your resort's money-back guarantee.

If you're headed to an all-inclusive resort, find out what that means, exactly. Have you paid for your lodging and food only? Are water sports and entertainment included? What about gratuities? Do you have to shell out for transportation to and from the airport?

Really Know Your Destination

If you're off to a foreign country, play the part of a diplomat. Learn some phrases in the native language. Don't expect everyone to speak English, and don't balk at the customs. If the food turns your stomach, don't chastise the locals for eating it. Remember, you're the foreigner here. Act as you would if you were a guest in someone's home, and you should return to your home soil relatively unscathed.

Don't Forget . . .

It's actually safer to use your credit cards (or traveler's checks) than to carry around huge wads of cash. The regular stipulations apply. Don't go wild charging everything just because you're on vacation, and keep track of how much you're spending. Be aware that you will need some cash, however, if you're planning on hitting the smaller inns and restaurants in foreign countries, many of which operate on a cash-only basis. Have your groom wear a money belt for the safekeeping of your coin.

Be sure to confirm your hotel reservations the week before you leave. There's nothing quite like dragging all your heavy luggage into a hotel lobby in some exotic locale, dreaming of a nice, long nap—only to find that you don't have a room. And there's not a vacant room on the island. If the room you thought you booked isn't the room you're being given, speak up. Ask for the manager on duty, and don't take no for an answer.

Once you arrive at your hotel, don't be afraid to complain to the management if the service or accommodations are not to your satisfaction. And don't wait until you're leaving. Most reputable hotels will go out of their way to rectify any problems as soon as possible, whether that means having your room cleaned again (the right way), or moving you to another room if possible, one that's not right next to the vending machines.

Eco-Tourism

After all of your careful vegan wedding planning, and the care you have taken in your life to respect life and the environment, consider making your honeymoon an eco-experience. Whether you call it eco-tourism, green travel, sustainable tourism, or green honeymoons, there are many shades of green, from green lodging to eco-adventure trips to volunteer vacations for your ultimate vacation. All of the green travel possibilities are based on the values and ideals of preserving, conserving, and protecting the natural and cultural environment of the locations you visit.

What's What?

Here are the definitions of several terms you may see while planning your honeymoon:

- **Ecotourism:** This word gets thrown around a lot in the travel industry, and many people try to take advantage of what it really means. The Ecotourism Society defines it as "responsible travel to natural areas which conserves the environment and improves the welfare of the local people." Unless your trip actually helps conserve and preserve, it is not a real eco-tour. The money you pay for your lodging and activities should go to the area and the people you visit, not into the pockets of some big corporation.

- **Adventure travel:** This is another term that is often misrepresented. It actually means an unusual experience that includes some level of risk or difficulty. Adventure travel may or may not be green. It will all depend on what you do and where you go. Backpacking in the mountains, rock climbing, and whitewater rafting can be green as long as you tread lightly and leave the natural locations unharmed.
- **Nature-based tourism:** This is a highly used phrase that can mean anything from camping in nature to viewing penguins from a ship to staying in a lodge in the middle of a tropical jungle. It is not necessarily green, although it could be.
- **Sustainable tourism:** This is a form of tourism that does not reduce resources and will ensure that future visitors will be able to enjoy the same experience you do. This means you are not disrupting or damaging the wildlife, natural habitat, or beauty of the area.
- **Responsible tourism:** These travels focus on leave-no-trace ethics. You want to preserve nature, not destroy it. A camping trip, hiking tour, even horseback riding along trails is fine as long as you leave the area as you found it.
- **Cultural tourism:** This is a trip that will have you interacting with and observing the native people of an area. You will be able to learn about their culture and participate in their activities, perhaps even live as they do. In simple ways, you participate in cultural tourism by shopping and eating at the local market or by learning about traditional dress and customs, maybe taking a pottery class from a local artisan.
- **Green tourism:** This term is often used along with or instead of "sustainable tourism" or "ecotourism," but it is most accurately described as tourism that includes any facility or activity that operates in an eco-friendly manner. Staying at a bed and breakfast that is powered by solar energy and uses only all-natural cleaning products and serves organic meals can be considered green tourism.
- **Multisport adventures:** While a sport vacation may not necessarily be green, it certainly can be. Those who operate outdoor recreational activities are often concerned about preserving nature and may have very green business practices.

- **Service trips/volunteer vacations:** These are trips you can take that will have you working for a good cause. The Sierra Club offers hands-on service trips for a wide variety of skills and physical levels. You can build and maintain trails, help archaeologists, repair meadows, and work in parks and wilderness areas. Some volunteer organizations only require you to pay for your transportation, while others require minimal fees for food and lodging. Most programs give you nights off and at least one day a week off to have time to explore the area and take in the sights and local culture.

Before You Commit

When you are looking for an area or location for your honeymoon, get the answers to these important questions before you make your choice:

❍ Will the money we spend go into the local economy? Will it help support the people and the natural elements in that location?

❍ Is the lodging location or tour company respectful of the local culture and environment? Is it active in conservation efforts?

❍ Are the activities we plan to do safe for the environment? Will they leave everything as we found it?

❍ Are we comfortable with the location? Does it represent our values and what we want in a honeymoon?

It all boils down to finding a honeymoon destination and experience that will be enjoyable and memorable for both of you. Before you start planning, discuss what you both want from your honeymoon. Is it romance and relaxation? Pampering and fun in the sun? Frolicking in the beauty of nature? A truly meaningful getaway that is enjoyable for you and helpful to others? Mix it up and blend the ideas together. There is nothing that says you can't have it all, even if you have to go to more than one destination. Once you decide what kind of trip you want to take, you can start looking for a destination and appropriate lodging.

Green Lodging

There are several types of green lodging available, and many locations are taking steps to become more eco-responsible. Some locations participate in extensive recycling programs, while others have implemented the use of renewable energy sources to provide power. Some have remodeled with environmentally friendly supplies, and other locations use all-natural cleaning products.

ALERT

The negative effects of tourism are taking a toll on the environment. Beaches are eroding, fragile ecosystems are being threatened, and carbon dioxide emissions from airplanes and automobiles are contributing to global warming. Almost 1 billion tourists travel around the globe every year.

Eco-Lodges

One green lodging choice is known as an eco-lodge. A real eco-lodge is set in a natural environment that allows visitors to experience the area's authentic local setting, cuisine, community, and culture. It is not really comfort based, and it may not offer many amenities—possibly not even such creature comforts as electricity or running water. It is all about nature and leaving the smallest impact possible on the natural setting. Some eco-lodges have no electricity, while others use only solar, wind, or other natural energy.

Eco-Resorts

An eco-resort blends the natural elements of an eco-lodge with luxury comforts such as electricity, running water, satellite television, wireless Internet, and even luxury spa treatments and activities. An eco-resort combines sustainability and comfort to create a fabulous green getaway.

Green Hotels

Green hotels are doing their best to be eco-friendly. Hotels, inns, and bed and breakfasts are earning the green label by incorporating eco-changes into their business. These hotels often incorporate vegan, vegetarian, and nonvegetarian meals of local, seasonal, and organic foods along with fair-trade coffees and teas. They take steps to reduce energy consumption as well as composting, recycling, and using environmentally friendly cleaning products.

Finding Eco-Friendly Lodging

What should you be looking for in a green hotel, inn, or B&B? Many locations are making changes from simple sustainable choices to extensive green renovations. The following are just some ways locations are becoming greener:

- Participating in recycling programs; having recycling stations in guest rooms or where guests have access to them
- Using all-natural cleaning supplies
- Offering organic, local, and fair-trade menus
- Installing low-flow, water-conserving showerheads, toilets, and faucets
- Using recycled paper products and paper-free invoicing and billing
- Providing reusable materials instead of single-use disposables
- Providing guests with bicycle rentals or carpooling/company shuttle bus transportation
- Building and remodeling with green materials
- Using low- or no-VOC (volatile organic compound) paint
- Providing bamboo, hemp, or organic cotton linens
- Using energy-efficient appliances, and sensors, and timers for thermostats, and CFL bulbs
- Powering with renewable energy such as solar or wind

Making the Trip

While everything seems to have been all about the wedding, now it is all about getting you to your ultimate destination. Once you and your fiancé make the decision regarding your destination, reserve it and begin making the necessary arrangements for the trip. To be sure you can relax and enjoy, there are some simple steps to take so that your home is safe and being cared for.

You are almost there . . . just a few more things to do:

○ Go to the bank—get money, traveler's checks, etc.
○ Double check travel advisories
○ Go through your packing list
○ Gather your travel documents
○ Make sure you have TSA-approved luggage locks
○ Book and/or confirm airport transportation
○ Make arrangements with your mom or maid of honor or drop off any rentals, ship your bouquet (to be preserved), and deliver your dress (to the preservationist)
○ Call the airline to check flights, restrictions on luggage and carry-ons, security alerts, seat reservations, and special meal requests
○ Confirm reservations with the hotel
○ Confirm the rental car

CHAPTER 20

Beyond the Wedding

Believe it or not, the day will come when you will wake up a married woman and no longer have a wedding to plan. That, however, does not mean you are off the hook. After all the months you spent planning, you must still dedicate a little more of your precious time to taking care of some remaining details like changing your name, writing thank-you notes, and maybe, even more importantly, establishing a vegan and green home as husband and wife. Oh, yeah, by the way . . . congratulations! Now go on and enjoy married life!

The Name Game

For years, you may have taken your own surname for granted, but faced with its possible loss, you may find yourself more attached to the name than you'd realized. This is the name you went through school with, the name you went to work with, the name everyone knows you by. It feels like a part of you. On the other hand, maybe your last name is ten syllables long, or no one can ever pronounce or spell it right, and you can't wait to get rid of it.

Options

When it comes time to change or not change your name, lucky for you, there are options. Here's the scoop on getting it done.

- Use your maiden name as your middle name and your husband's as your last. So if Julia Andrews married Joseph Nelson, she'd be Julia Andrews Nelson.
- Hyphenate the two last names: Julia Andrews-Nelson. This means that the two separate last names are now joined to make one name (kind of like a marriage). You keep your regular middle name, but saying your full name can be a mouthful: Julia Marie Andrews-Nelson.
- Take your husband's name legally, but use your maiden name professionally. In everyday life and social situations, you'd use your married name, but in the office, you'd use the same name you always had.
- Hyphenate both your and your husband's last names: Julia Andrews-Nelson and Richard Andrews-Nelson.

Make It Legal

Before you can make any official changes to your name, you will need to have your official marriage license. Once that is in hand, you can download forms from the Internet (or pick them up, request them via mail or phone) and get going on this momentous change. You will need a new Social Security card and a legally valid form of identification, usually a driver's license.

One easy way to tackle this task is with a name-change kit. These kits are widely available and provide the proper forms and information you need to legally change your name. Each state has its own requirements, so be sure to purchase a kit that is customized for your state.

NAME-CHANGE DOCUMENT CHECKLIST
- ○ Bank accounts (savings, checking, 401(k) plans, investment accounts, etc.)
- ○ Car registrations
- ○ Credit cards
- ○ Driver's license
- ○ Employment records
- ○ Insurance policies
- ○ Internal Revenue Service records
- ○ Leases
- ○ Passport
- ○ Pension plan records
- ○ Post office listings
- ○ Property titles
- ○ School records or alumni listings
- ○ Social Security
- ○ Stock certificates
- ○ Utility and telephone information
- ○ Voter registration
- ○ Will

Thank You! Thank You!

For better or worse, thank-you notes are one rule of etiquette that's here to stay. While everyone appreciates the gift, writing thank-you notes does not generally rank up there as a favorite task of anyone's. Ironically, in today's world of instant communication, you are still expected to send a handwritten personalized thank-you note every time you receive a gift, and your friends and family do appreciate the sentiment.

As soon as you receive a gift, you should send out a thank-you note. As hard as it will be considering the many notes you'll be writing, try to be warm and personal. Always mention the gift, and, if possible, how you and your fiancé will be using it. This small touch will prevent people from feeling that you just sent them a form letter (which, by the way, is completely unacceptable, no matter how busy you are). When sending notes for gifts you receive before the wedding, sign your maiden name.

What to Say

Thank-you notes from any shower gifts should be (or should have been!) sent within a few weeks of receiving the gift. For wedding gifts received prior to the wedding, it is perfectly acceptable to send thank-you notes as soon as you receive the gift. Just be sure to sign your maiden name to any thank-you cards written before you're married. As for gifts received at or after the wedding, make an effort to write your thank yous as soon as possible, such as within a month or two.

Really, thank-you notes are pretty simple. Here is what to include:

❍ Mention the gift
❍ Make a brief statement about how you plan to use it
❍ Thank the guest for their generosity

Here are a couple of samples to help get you started.

Thank-You Note for a Wedding Gift

Dear Lynn and Dennis,
Thank you so much for the gorgeous set of bamboo cutting boards. We really look forward to inviting you to our home very soon to enjoy a lovely meal. Those cutting boards will be of great use in our kitchen. Thank you for taking the time to shop at our favorite store and support an ethical business. We are so glad you were able to be with us at our wedding.
Fondly,
Julia

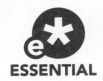

ESSENTIAL

Thank-You Note for a Monetary Gift

Dear Barbara and Art,

Thank you so much for the generous gift. It will truly help us in purchasing green and cruelty-free kitchenware for our new home. We appreciate your thoughtfulness and support of our vegan wedding. We are so glad you were able to be with us at our wedding.

Fondly,

Julia

Returns and Exchanges

What if someone sends you a lava lamp along with a fringed lampshade? Your first instinct, assuming your decorating tastes are in a completely different vein, might be to immediately throw the lamp out, burn it, or exchange it for something else. But it's not as simple as that. The people who bought you that gift did so with the best of intentions, spending a good deal of their time, energy, and money on you. Imagine how hurt they'd be if they visited your house a week after the wedding, expecting the lamp to hold a place of honor, only to find that you'd exchanged it for some napkin rings.

The best thing you can do to avoid this awkward situation is to wait until about a month after the wedding to exchange any unwanted or duplicate gifts. Some couples display all of the gifts they've received somewhere in their home in the days before the wedding; people who visit you at that time are likely to look for their gifts and even ask your opinions about them. After the wedding, when everything is put away in its proper place, guests are less likely to make an issue out of their gifts. Waiting to return or exchange gifts is also a good policy regarding gifts you receive at the reception.

If you receive a damaged gift, try to track down the retailer who sold the item. If this item didn't come from your registry, you may need to let the giver know that the gift was delivered in a less-than-perfect condition. You may be directed to the store where the purchase was made, or the giver may offer to exchange the gift for you. She may still have the receipt, and in any event, she's in a much better position than you are to deal with the store. She's the customer, she's the one who spent her money there, and she's the one who is going to get the concessions she's looking for from the store manager.

Oh, the Memories!

Two very sentimental items from a bride's wedding day are her gown and her bouquet. Whether or not you choose to keep these is entirely up to you. If you do wish to preserve these special mementos, check into your options early on, so that your wishes can become a reality.

ESSENTIAL

After having planned and participated in this momentous once-in-a-lifetime occasion, you must now go back to work and your "normal" life. Realize it takes time to adjust. Be patient and share your feelings with your husband. To ease the adjustment, find a reason to celebrate—just a little—on your monthly anniversaries.

Parting with the Gown

Keeping or not keeping your gown is a very personal decision. Whatever you decide, the gown needs to be cleaned. Here are a few ways brides part with their gowns.

- Sell the gown, either through a local consignment shop or on the Internet. Keep in mind this may not be an easy process, as it has been altered and worn. In that case, a wedding gown is like a car . . . once you drive it off the lot, the value drops significantly, so don't expect to get a huge return on your investment.
- Donate your gown to a local charitable thrift shop. The proceeds from the sale will help whichever charity the thrift shop is affiliated with.
- Donating your gown to a local or national organization that sells gently used (and new) gowns across the country with proceeds helping make wishes come true for breast cancer patients.
- Donate your gown to a fashion school, local college, or high school.

Keeping the Gown

On the other hand, if you want to keep and treasure this precious garment "forever," professional gown preservation is a must. Prior to the wedding, you should look into preserving; though not ideal, it really isn't too late to do it once you return from the honeymoon.

With preserving, the gown will be cleaned, removing visible and nonvisible stains, and minor tears and damages as well as beading and lacework will be repaired. Look for a gown preservation company that uses pH neutral, acid-free paper and containers. You should also be able to remove your gown from the box to inspect it. Finally, be sure to work with a company that guarantees their services.

The Bouquet

Many brides choose to preserve their bridal bouquet as a memento of the wedding. Whether this is done professionally or is more of a DIY project does not really matter. If this is an important item to you and keeping it is something you have your heart set on, do a little research to ensure you are going to get the outcome you desire.

If professionally preserving your bouquet is out of the question or out of the budget, look to some of the following DIY alternatives to preserve these special flowers.

Pressing

This is one of the most popular means of bouquet preservation. The steps to successfully pressing your bouquet are as follows but note that the process works best when it's started soon after the wedding because the flowers have had less time to wilt. If you ask real nice and promise to return the favor, you might just be able to convince your maid of honor to do it while you're on your honeymoon.

- Take a picture of your bouquet; you'll need it to refer to later.
- Take the bouquet apart (and that's no typo).
- Place the separate flowers in the pages of heavy books, between sheets of blank white paper (warning: if you neglect to cushion with blank paper, ink from the book's pages will ruin the flowers).
- Keep flowers in books for two to six weeks, depending on their size (hint: the bigger the flower, the more time it will need).
- When the flowers look ready, glue them onto a mounting board in an arrangement that closely resembles the original bouquet in the photo.
- Place the board in a picture frame.
- Hang wherever your heart desires.

Hanging/Drying

As with pressing, the earlier you start the process, the more successful it's likely to be. Here are the steps:

- Snap a photo for future reference.
- Take the bouquet apart.
- Hang the flowers upside down to dry, thereby preventing drooping and keeping the flowers' shape intact (some color may be lost in the drying process, but this can be avoided if the flowers are hung in a dark room).
- When the flowers are completely dry, spray them with a finishing spray for protection.
- Reassemble flowers to match the photo.

Creating a Vegan Home

As a vegan, your health and the world around you are extremely important to you. And what is more important than where you live? The space you live in and surround yourself with is a reflection of you, your life, and your beliefs. This is also a time of transition and changes. The answers may not be apparent right away, and there may have to be some frank discussions about the type of home you will establish.

Making Decisions

Now that you are married, there will be transitions in your life, but how much of a transition there is in your home is dependent on a few things:

- Are you both vegan?
- Will your home be a vegan home?
- If you are not both vegan, what choices and compromise are each of you willing to make to keep the other happy and your home harmonious?
- If you were already living together, are you happy with your current home and health, or do you want to make changes to create a greener home?

Vegan Transitions

Even if you lived together prior to the wedding, it is different once you are married. It is hard to explain, but it is true. There is a transition into life as a married couple. If both of you are vegans, the transition to a married couple living in a single household will be smoother. If only one of you is a vegan and now you are joining your households, you both need to be willing to listen to each other and compromise and look for solutions to make your home a happy place.

You may need to establish which pots and pans, dishes, utensils, and storage containers are for vegan meals only and which for nonvegan meals. You may even wish to designate shelves in the refrigerator and pantry for the same purposes. Each of you needs to realize there are reasons the other has chosen to live the way they do.

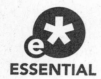

If the household is mixed with vegans and nonvegans, consider making it a rule that shared items such as toothpaste, cleaning supplies, and linens are vegan items.

A Vegan Home

Chances are good that if you and your hubby are both vegan, the furnishings, accessories, and essentials you bring to your home together are vegan. It is easy to tell if something is leather or suede, but some items are not as noticeable. The inclusion of animal products into finishes on furnishings and trimmings is high and invasive.

Keep It, Toss It

Sometime as you combine households, you will discover that one or both of you have a seemingly benign yet nonvegan item. What to do!? You can donate it right away and get it out of the home, but what if there are no funds to replace it? Many couples find it acceptable to use the piece (assuming it is an essential item, and the offending issue is something like a furniture finish) until it breaks or wears out or they can afford to replace it with a vegan item.

Twelve-Month Wedding Planning Checklist

After the dust settles from the whirlwind of excitement and celebrating with family and friends, there are some things you'll have to do to actually get married. Depending upon the type and size wedding you decide to have, you may have lots to do or tons to do. In any event, the following schedule should give you a general idea of what has to be done, and when you should do it.

TEN TO TWELVE MONTHS

- ○ Select engagement ring
- ○ Insure ring
- ○ Announce engagement
- ○ Set date
- ○ Attend engagement party
- ○ Hire wedding planner
- ○ Draft preliminary guest list
- ○ Draft budget
- ○ Begin bridal registry
- ○ Determine style and formality
- ○ Research ceremony venue
- ○ Research reception venue
- ○ Begin researching, interviewing, and hiring vendors
- ○ Set up wedding website

EIGHT TO TEN MONTHS

- ○ Select wedding party
- ○ Select ceremony venue
- ○ Select reception venue
- ○ Shop for gown
- ○ Book caterer (if necessary)
- ○ Book entertainment
- ○ Book photographer
- ○ Book videographer
- ○ Order Save-the-Date cards

SIX TO EIGHT MONTHS

- ○ Order wedding gown
- ○ Book florist
- ○ Book hair stylist
- ○ Book makeup artist
- ○ Order wedding cake

- ○ Hire officiate
- ○ Secure rentals
- ○ Organize travel accommodations for guests
- ○ Organize accommodations for wedding night (and night before)
- ○ Schedule engagement photo session (after hiring photographer)
- ○ Research wedding invitations
- ○ Research honeymoon destinations and check travel advisories
- ○ Finalize remaining vendor commitments
- ○ Book parking attendants
- ○ Order bridesmaids' dresses
- ○ Research other stationery needs (menu cards, place cards, ceremony programs)

FOUR TO SIX MONTHS

- ○ Mail Save-the-Date cards
- ○ Select formalwear for the groom and men
- ○ Have mothers shop for attire
- ○ Plan rehearsal dinner
- ○ Plan prewedding and postwedding parties
- ○ Finalize guest list
- ○ Order wedding invitations and announcements
- ○ Order invitations for rehearsal dinner, and prewedding and postwedding parties
- ○ Hire calligrapher for invitations and place cards
- ○ Book honeymoon
- ○ Get passports (if necessary)

TWO TO FOUR MONTHS

- ○ Select wedding day transportation
- ○ Shop for wedding bands

- ○ Research marriage license requirements
- ○ Research and select a seamstress for alterations
- ○ Select wedding favors
- ○ Determine reception menu
- ○ Finalize cake flavors and design
- ○ Shop for bridal accessories (lingerie, jewelry, headpiece/veil, etc.)
- ○ Shop for bridesmaids' accessories (jewelry, shoes, purses)
- ○ Develop preliminary itinerary for wedding day
- ○ Verify gown delivery date
- ○ Address and assemble invitations
- ○ Have invitations weighed at post office, buy postage for invitation and response envelopes
- ○ Confirm delivery dates for wedding gown and bridesmaids' dresses

ONE TO TWO MONTHS

- ○ Mail invitations (six to eight weeks)
- ○ Shop for thank-you gifts (attendants, parents, etc.)
- ○ Prepare shot list for videographer and photographer
- ○ Make arrangements for preserving bridal bouquet
- ○ Make arrangements for preserving bridal gown
- ○ Have wedding day hair and makeup preview
- ○ Finalize rehearsal-dinner plans
- ○ Send rehearsal-dinner invitations
- ○ Finalize ceremony details
- ○ Finalize reception details

- ○ Finalize musical selections with entertainment
- ○ Attend dress fittings/alterations
- ○ Prepare wedding announcement for newspaper
- ○ Attend wedding showers
- ○ Purchase wedding accessories (guestbook/pen, ring pillow, etc.)
- ○ Schedule final beauty appointments

ONE MONTH

- ○ Get marriage license
- ○ Finalize itinerary with vendors and ceremony/reception locations
- ○ Begin seating plan for reception
- ○ Pick up wedding bands
- ○ Schedule final gown fittings and confirm pick-up date
- ○ Write thank-you notes (for any wedding gifts already received)
- ○ Break in your wedding shoes
- ○ Begin finalizing wedding day itinerary

TWO WEEKS

- ○ Final guest count due to caterer/reception location
- ○ Call guests who have not responded
- ○ Confirm rehearsal-dinner guest count
- ○ Begin packing for honeymoon
- ○ Make final payments to vendors (payments due between now up to wedding day)
- ○ Finalize seating chart and send seating/place cards to calligrapher
- ○ Prepare a Bridal Emergency Kit

ONE WEEK

- ○ Pick up gown
- ○ Attend final grooming appointments
- ○ Call/e-mail venues and all vendors to finalize arrangements, delivery times, etc.
- ○ Attend bachelor/bachelorette parties
- ○ Arrange to have mail/package delivery stopped (during your honeymoon)
- ○ Attend bridal luncheon

TWO TO THREE DAYS

- ○ Pick up tuxedoes for groom and men
- ○ Cut checks for remaining vendor payments
- ○ Prepare vendor tips
- ○ Drop off wedding accessories at venue or to wedding planner
- ○ Pack bag for the wedding day

ONE DAY

- ○ Attend ceremony rehearsal and distribute wedding day itinerary
- ○ Deliver remaining accessories to wedding planner, church coordinator, etc.
- ○ Attend rehearsal dinner
- ○ Present attendants with their gifts at the rehearsal dinner
- ○ Go to bed early—get your rest!

THE WEDDING DAY

- ○ Give vendor tips and payments to best man or wedding planner
- ○ Marry the man you love, and have a great day!

POST WEDDING

- ○ Send bouquet for preservation
- ○ Send gown for cleaning and preservation
- ○ Complete and mail thank-you cards
- ○ Thank your vendors (phone call and/or note)
- ○ Thank your parents and attendants (phone call and/or note)
- ○ Change name

Vegan Resources

We do not endorse any of the following sites over any other vegan/green sites or products. It is the responsibility of the bride and groom or whoever is making the purchase/contact to do due diligence when purchasing or hiring.

Vegan General and Lifestyle Resources

Chef AJ
Plant-based whole-food chef and author of *Unprocessed*
www.chefajshealthykitchen.com
www.eatunprocessed.com
www.healthytasteofla.com

Eat Locally Resources
www.eatwellguide.org
www.localharvest.org
www.sustainabletable.org

Food News
www.foodnews.org

Happy Cow
www.happycow.net

The Organic Report
www.theorganicreport.com

The Organic Wine Company
www.theorganicwinecompany.com

Peta (People for the Ethical Treatment of Animals)
www.Peta.org

Raw Guru
www.rawguru.com

Soy Stache
www.soystache.com/vegorg.htm

Vegan Action
www.vegan.org

Vegan Baking
www.veganbaking.net

Vegan Coach
www.vegancoach.com

Vegan Essentials
www.veganessentials.com

VegNews **(Printed and online publication)**
www.vegnews.com

Vegan Paradise
www.veganparadise.com

Veg Source
www.vegsource.com

VegWeb.com
www.vegweb.com

Vegan Wine Guide
www.vegans.frommars.org/wine

The Vegan Voice
www.theveganvoice.org

Your Vegan Guide
www.bestveganguide.com

Vegan and Green Weddings

Ethical Weddings
A UK-based resource that has advice and vendor listings for all over the world
www.ethicalweddings.com

Portovert
www.portovert.com

Rose Pedals Vegan Weddings
Features real vegan weddings and resources
www.rosepedalsveganweddings.com

Vegan Nutritionista
All-encompassing vegan site, but has a series of wedding-planning articles
www.vegan-nutritionista.com

Recycling Information

Recycling Markets
www.recyclingmarkets.net

The National Recycling Coalition
www.nrc-recycle.org

Earth 911
www.earth911.org

Charitable Giving

I Do Foundation
www.idofoundation.org

Charity Guide
www.charityguide.org

Network for Good
www.networkforgood.org

Charity
www.charity.com

Just Give
www.justgive.org

Give
www.give.org

Habitat for Humanity
www.habitat.org

The World Wildlife Fund
www.justgive.org

The Nature Conservancy
www.nature.org

The National Wildlife Federation
www.nwf.org

Index

We Have EVERYTHING® on Anything!

The Everything® list spans a wide range of subjects, with more than 500 titles covering 25 different categories:

Business	History	Reference
Careers	Home Improvement	Religion
Children's Storybooks	Everything Kids	Self-Help
Computers	Languages	Sports & Fitness
Cooking	Music	Travel
Crafts and Hobbies	New Age	Wedding
Education/Schools	Parenting	Writing
Games and Puzzles	Personal Finance	
Health	Pets	